THE ENERGY WITHIN

THE
ENERGY
WITHIN

The Science Behind every Oriental Therapy from Acupuncture to Yoga

RICHARD M. CHIN
M.D., O.M.D.

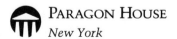 PARAGON HOUSE
New York

First edition, 1992

Published in the United States by

Paragon House
90 Fifth Avenue
Copyright © 1992 by Richard M. Chin

Library of Congress Cataloging-in-Publication Data

Chin, Richard,
    The energy within : the science behind every oriental therapy
from acupuncture to yoga / Richard M. Chin.—1st ed.
      p. cm.
    Includes index.
    ISBN 1–55778–349–7 : $12.95
     1. Alternative medicine. 2. Bioenergetics. 3. Holistic
medicine. 4. Medicine, Oriental. I. Title.
  R733.C484 1992
  610'.95—dc20   91–24989
                                            CIP

Printed in the United States of America.

CONTENTS

	INTRODUCTION	vii
Chapter One	WHAT IS ENERGY?	I
Chapter Two	WHAT DOES ENERGETICS HAVE TO DO WITH ME?	14
Chapter Three	HOW ENERGY WORKS IN YOUR BODY	40
Chapter Four	ENERGETICS: BODY, MIND, AND SPIRIT	89
Chapter Five	MAXIMUM ENERGY FOR LIFE	126
Chapter Six	THIRTY MINUTES, THIRTY DAYS TO MAXIMUM ENERGY	150
	AFTERWORD	199
	APPENDIX	201

INTRODUCTION

ENERGY IS the basis of all life. It comprises and links everything in the universe, from the stars in the sky to the atoms that make up those stars—all we can see and all we cannot. As parts of the universe, we, too, are comprised of energy. In fact, our inner energy is simply a reflection of the greater play of energies in the universe as a whole. And when this inner energy becomes unbalanced or stops flowing, we experience illness or disease.

Energetics is the science of understanding and harmonizing this universal energy. Energetic medicine is based on relating the basic principles behind energetics to the energy that flows throughout our own minds and bodies—and on keeping this energy moving and in balance in order to prevent illness and create a maximum state of health. Understanding how the fundamentals of energetics relate to you and the world around you is the first step to acquiring the maximum energy that accompanies a balanced life.

The world's scientific community agrees that energy

comprises all things. But when it comes to applying this same idea to the human body, Eastern and Western medicine hold extremely divergent views. While Eastern medicine is based on balancing our internal energy, Western medicine has yet to fully agree that a distinct energy system exists within our bodies at all.

Both Eastern and Western health care have their own strengths and weaknesses. Eastern medicine is described as having a "holistic" approach to medicine because it treats body and mind as a single entity. But I do not believe true holistic medicine, *total* health care, will be practiced until East and West accept each other's strengths while also accepting each other's differences. In fact, Eastern and Western medicine often reach the same conclusions, but they get there by vastly different means. Each culture has much to learn from the other.

As a physician with both Eastern and Western medical degrees, I have written this book from the Western point of view in order to make some basic Eastern concepts accessible to Western readers. When studying anything, oftentimes only a slight change in perspective allows us to see something astoundingly new—and to learn that much more about ourselves and about life itself. Studying how the human body works from both the Eastern and Western perspectives has allowed me to gain a few insights into each health care system that I would not otherwise have attained. I have tried to include as many of these insights as possible in this book.

As we head toward the twenty-first century, I believe physicians worldwide will begin to agree that the human organism is actually a matrix of interacting multidimensional energy fields. New methods of faster, safer diagnosis will become available as we start to realize that, via our own natural energy, we have the power to diagnose and heal illness even more effectively than the sophisticated machines we have created—and without harmful side effects. We must continue to study this power scientifically so that energetic healing methods may be further developed and integrated into current health care systems around the globe.

But while these changes may take many years to occur, this book can help you learn to take control of your own health care right now by learning how to develop and control your energy system. Since the time of the classical sages of ancient China, thousands of years ago, layers of myth have surrounded energetics, leading many people to believe that it is based on magic as opposed to science. I hope this book will help to eliminate this misunderstanding. Energetics is a very complex science, almost as complex as the mysterious life force it seeks to understand. After thirty years of studying it, I am still learning. My goal in writing this book is to leave you with a solid grasp of the basic principles of energetics, and show you how they can be used to maintain the delicate natural balance of energy that governs your health and well-being.

This book will guide you, step-by-step, on an incredible journey to the essence of your being. You must start the journey by becoming aware of the different forms energy takes, both around you and within you. You will learn about the mysterious properties that make up your life energy and, by performing a few simple exercises, you will learn how to actually feel it flowing within your body. You will understand the three levels of energy that comprise your body, mind, and spirit, and find out how they coexist in harmony—and what can happen when they become unbalanced. You will also learn different ways to keep all your different energies balanced and flowing properly. Once you become aware of the power of your own energy you can begin to develop it, and start to accomplish things you may never have thought yourself capable of. There is extraordinary potential within you. The power of your own energy is limited only by the amount of time and effort you are willing to devote to developing it. This book will help you begin your journey.

Richard M. Chin, M.D., O.M.D.

THE ENERGY WITHIN

Chapter One

WHAT IS ENERGY?

Wʜᴀᴛ ɪs energy? This question has intrigued scientists and philosophers for centuries, because to understand the essence of energy is to understand the essence of life itself. So what is energy? Is it the sun you feel warming your body? The gasoline you put in your car? The electricity you use to run a vacuum cleaner? The answer to all three questions is yes. These are all just different forms of the same universal energy. Where and how this primordial energy was created has always been life's great mystery, a question answered by imaginative myths and legends in almost every culture. We still do not know how this source of energy was created, but we are learning more and more about how energy works in our world. Understanding the mysterious laws that govern the limitless manifestations of energy is what the science of energetics is all about.

To understand the basic principles behind energetics, it is helpful to compare three views on universal energy: today's Western, "scientific" view, the ancient Chinese tradition, and the view from ancient India.

THE WESTERN TRADITION

The "scientific" view of energetics is the one currently accepted by most of the Western world, and by most scientists all over the world, as the explanation for the beginning of the universe and the role of energy within it. This view is based on the big bang theory, which holds that about twenty billion years ago the universe was created in one powerful explosion that sent elemental particles scattering into space. About one-third of these particles carried a positive charge, one-third a negative charge, and the remaining third a neutral charge. As the universe continued to expand outward after this explosion, a tremendous amount of heat was released. By the time the universe was about one million years old it cooled down, and these particles started to group together into atoms and molecules, much as water will crystalize at lower temperatures to form ice. According to the currently accepted view, as the universe continued to cool down, these groups of elemental particles formed the primary elements of all matter.

Two basic tenets of Western scientific thought, the laws concerning the conservation of matter and the conservation of energy, say that matter and energy can be neither created nor destroyed; they can only change into other forms of matter or energy, respectively. These laws scientifically established the idea that both matter and energy move in cycles without beginning or end. Later Albert Einstein proposed, with his famous formula $E = mc^2$, that energy *is* an expression of matter and vice versa, and that the potential molecular energy contained within matter can be released. (The confirmation of this theory led to the creation of the atomic bomb.) So even though you cannot directly observe the moving atomic particles that comprise matter, Albert Einstein proved to the Western world that everything in the universe, from the car you drive to the chair you are sitting on to your own body, is just a different form of energy.

Many people believe that this scientific approach must represent the most advanced view on energy, because the West is much more technologically advanced than other parts of the world. But although technology has provided the Western world with many important scientific advantages, when it comes to understanding the essence of energy as the essence of life itself, this approach has proven futile. Scientists use technology to analyze things by breaking them down into smaller and smaller parts. This method of investigation often yields important insights, but it cannot be used to understand energy as the essence of life. I recall having heard this idea best expressed in a lecture by Dr. Nguyen Van Nghi, a man considered to be the grandfather of Oriental medicine in Europe. He said the modern methods Western science uses to investigate energy—to discover it—are all fantasies, for once you strip this mysterious life force down to its barest components, you lose it altogether. Energy, the essence of life, cannot be isolated.

The power of technology lies in the way it uses and manipulates energy, in the way it sometimes *controls* energy. But you must understand its limitations. Technology cannot stop hurricanes, tornadoes, earthquakes, or other natural phenomena. It can only warn us of their approach so that we can protect ourselves. We can use technology to harness the power of energy, but not to solve the mysteries of the essence of that power. Technology will never allow us to actually control the winds, though it can help us learn how to let them carry us where we want to go.

Now compare this modern view of energy to two of the most ancient views on record: the Chinese and Indian traditions.

THE ANCIENT CHINESE TRADITION

Like today's scientific or Western view on energy, the ancient Chinese tradition also holds that the universe began with a single universal energy source. This source of all energy is said to represent non-being, and is the neutral essence of life. It is the beginningless beginning, the mover and the movement—in short, it is everything.

One of the basic differences between the Eastern and Western views on energy is that Eastern philosophies are not really concerned with *why* the universe is as it is or how it came into being. They simply accept the existence of the universe as it is. Western thought is more focused on the cause or creator behind it. According to the Chinese or Taoist philosophy, the world as we know it comes from a "great void." This void is made up of *qi* (pronounced "chee"), the Chinese term for energy. (This term is also frequently spelled *chi*. Because Chinese words are romanized in different ways, there are often many alternate spellings for basic energetic terms.) The things around us, including our own bodies, are made up of this *qi*. The Chinese see the universe as constantly changing, but they do not look for the answers to the mysteries of life *behind* this changing universe, but instead *within* the patterns and order of it.

According to the Chinese tradition, while all manifestations of *qi* depend on change, the primary source of *qi* never changes. From it all creation arises and to it all creation returns. This, again, coincides with the Western theory that matter and energy are essentially the same thing and can neither be created nor destroyed— both simply contain the potential to assume different forms.

From this primary state of *qi* comes the next stage of *yin* and *yang* as represented by the *tai chi* symbol (see figure 1). Understanding the significance of this symbol will provide you with an overall understanding of how the Chinese view the order of the universe. The circle representing all of being is divided into the black *yin* and white *yang* areas. *Yin* and *yang* represent the essence of life—conflict and interdependency. They do not represent separate, opposing elements; to the contrary, they symbolize that nothing can exist in and of itself. Everything exists in relation to everything else, and can only be understood within the context of this relationship. Therefore, you cannot change one part of the universe without affecting the entire universe. Although modern physics, too, currently presents a holistic view of the universe, much of the remainder of Western culture is just starting to accept this theory.

So the meaning of the *tai chi* symbol is not discerned by taking it apart, but instead by looking at it in its totality. The symbol shows us that there are no such things as opposites, per se, just two ways of seeing the same thing—and each of these two aspects is always in the process of becoming the other. We cannot understand what something is without understanding all it is not. For example, you would not be able to understand daytime without knowing what nighttime was, or hot without cold, or a negative charge without a positive charge. In fact, as soon as you create one aspect, you instantly create the other in order to understand it. This idea is further represented by the dots in the symbol, which show us that *yin* is within *yang* and vice versa.

Yin and *yang* are linked by the relationship each side has to the other. Each aspect continually works to control, balance, and harmonize the other. They represent the constant give-and-take relationship that is life activity itself, thereby establishing a process where the potential for movement arises. *Qi* constantly passes back and forth between them. Life is based on this potential: the flow of electricity between positive and negative poles, the contraction and extension of the muscles in your body, and so on.

Although *yin* is the phase of energy associated with negative, contractive, and receptive characteristics, and *yang* is associated with positive, expansive, and outgoing characteristics, the terms do not necessarily correspond to any specific forces. Life is based on the movement of *qi*, so in order to sustain life, *qi* must keep moving. But in order for movement to occur there must be something else to move to. Therefore, all things must have at least two primary aspects, here described as *yin* and *yang*, in order for life to continue to exist.

CHINESE TRADITION

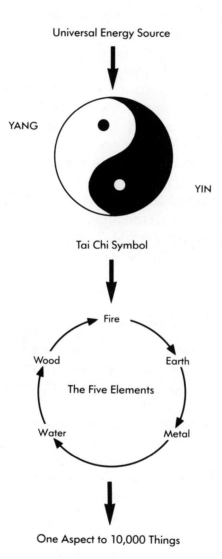

Universal Energy Source

YANG

YIN

Tai Chi Symbol

The Five Elements

Fire

Earth

Metal

Water

Wood

One Aspect to 10,000 Things

According to the Chinese tradition, *qi* first arises from a primary energy source and then separates into the polarities of *yin* and *yang*. It then further intensifies, gradually becoming denser and more physical to form the "five phases": earth, water, fire, wood, and metal, from which all things are made. (The five phases will be discussed in greater detail in chapter 3.) This process can be compared to the workings of a transformer, which steps down intense forms of energy into less intense, slower currents of energy. Everything in the physical world, including our own bodies, thoughts, and emotions, are expressions of these lower stages of *qi*. The *qi* moves in *yin* and *yang* cycles and through the five phases to form all the things that make up both our internal and external world. This transformation is described in an old Chinese saying as "the one aspect to ten thousand things."

THE INDIAN TRADITION

Just as there are striking similarities between the Western scientific view on energy and the ancient Chinese view, there are concepts which both these traditions share with the ancient view from India. In the Indian tradition, too, there is a single supreme source of all energy, called *brahmon*. From *brahmon* arises all of consciousness and *prana*—the Indian term for life energy—and to it all must return (see figure 2).

Although *brahmon* is the primary source of all life, it has two distinct aspects: *purusha* and *prakrita*. *Purusha* is the Indian term meaning "conscious potential." While *purusha* itself has no polarity, it holds the poten-

INDIAN TRADITION

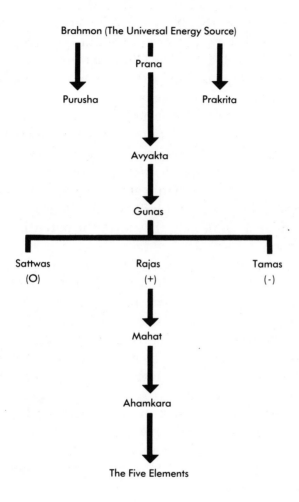

Brahmon (The Universal Energy Source)

Prana

Purusha · · · · · · Prakrita

Avyakta

Gunas

Sattwas · · · · · · Rajas · · · · · · Tamas
(O) · · · · · · · · · · (+) · · · · · · · · · · (-)

Mahat

Ahamkara

The Five Elements

Fire   Earth   Water   Air   Ether

tial for all polarity and all manifestations of *prana*. All of life's possibilities are contained within this neutral core. *Purusha* is the DNA within every cell—the instructions for how the *prana* should be directed and what form it will take. The Chinese term for this mysterious force representing the presence of a "higher intelligence" is *li* (pronounced "lee").

Prakrita, the second aspect of *brahmon*, relates to the creative impulses. It contains the potential source of *prana* behind actual creation, the vital impulse to bring non-being to being. While *purusha* contains the plans for all the forms or manifestations *prana* will take, *prakrita* is the power that brings these plans into being. So together, as *brahmon*, they form the potential for all of creation.

From *brahmon* comes the *avyahta* level of *prana*, which is similar to the Chinese *tai chi* stage. Here, the potential for polarity relationships latent in *purusha* takes form through the three *gunas*, which are similar to the Chinese concept of *yin* and *yang*. *Rajas* is the positive or *yang* aspect of the balance of energy. It represents a centrifugal force, moving outward from a center. *Tamas* is the negative or *yin* phase. Working both with and against *rajas*, it is the contractive, centripetal force. *Sattvas* is the neutral field which allows for the movement of *prana* and represents the balanced aspect of all polarity relationships, as does the *tai chi* symbol when seen as a whole.

Sattvas, *rajas*, and *tamas*, like *yin* and *yang*, set up polarity relationships that are inherent in every aspect of our lives and in all things around us. According to the Indian view, without the *gunas*, no polarities or conflicting forces could exist, so no movement of *prana* could take place, and life as we know it would not exist.

The remaining levels of *prana* are more detailed than in the Chinese view as they condense to form the matter that comprises all things. From the *gunas* arise the next level of *prana*, called *mahat*, or the cosmic intellect. When an individual's *prana* reaches this stage, usually through meditation, there is an awareness of the wholeness of existence. Although there is a cosmic knowledge of the oneness of all things, there exists simultaneously a subtle feeling of separation from *brahmon*.

The next level of *prana* intensification is called *ahamkara*, or the state of ego consciousness. At *ahamkara*, the separation experienced at *mahat* is deepened and the ego is experienced as separate from the world around it. The individual's energy has moved so far from *brahmon* that conscious contact with the universal energy source is lost, and ego arises. This is the level of existence man is essentially "trapped" in. Both *mahat* and *ahamkara* are also known as the causal or astral planes of existence.

From here *prana* moves into physical forms and is manifested as the five elements. Although both the Chinese and Indian views include fire, earth, and water as three of the five basic manifestations of energy, the Indian tradition adds the elements air and ether rather than the Chinese phases of wood and metal. The five elements complete the process that leads from the source of all energy to physical matter. As in the Chinese system, it is *prana*, or vital energy, which moves through the five elements to bring forth all of creation.

Even though we still do not know how the primary source of energy or *qi* or *prana* really came into existence, we are constantly learning more about *how* it exists. What is really fascinating is that of these theories, developed centuries apart in various parts of the globe and apparently so different, are *all basically in agreement* (much more so, in fact, than we can discuss in this chapter; that would require another book). They are just three different ways of saying the same things:

- Energy, despite its limitless manifestations, all comes from one universal source.
- Movement of energy is the basis of all life. In order for energy to move it must have an inherent polarity relationship; that is, it must have something or somewhere to move to.
- Matter is an expression of energy and vice versa. It can neither be created nor destroyed, only transformed into another form of energy.
- All things are manifestations of energy, including us; that is, all things are essentially "living" things in that energy flows through them, despite our inability to observe this phenomenon directly. The difference between what we describe as "animate" and "inanimate" is only the result of our own illusions.

Whether you ascribe to the Western, scientific viewpoint or the Chinese or Indian traditions, whether you use the terms positive and negative, *yin* and *yang*, or *rajas*, *tamas*, and *sattvas*, the same principles are being repeated again and again. All describe relationships that establish the potential for the flow of energy, for the creation and continuation of life.

All views on energy, from the most ancient to the most modern, share the same basic premise: that the world is comprised of energy flowing down from a primary source to become all things. The energy may be "directed" to take the form of an elephant, or electricity, or any of the endless variety of manifestations in between. Everyone agrees that the world around us is not what it seems to be. And so, after countless hours of research and "startling" new discoveries, twentieth-century science is finally learning what the ancient Eastern philosophies and traditions have known for ten thousand years.

Chapter Two

WHAT DOES ENERGETICS HAVE TO DO WITH ME?

THE ENERGY that exists within the universe is the same energy that exists within ourselves. It can be difficult to comprehend the existence of things you cannot see, and you cannot see your energy. You can, however, learn to actually *feel* it. But before you can do this, you must "suspend your disbelief" long enough to begin the work to find it. This chapter will get you started.

Although today's Western, scientific theory and the ancient Eastern traditions all agree that everything in the universe is made up of energy, they came to this similar understanding in very different ways. Whereas Western science developed its theory of the workings of the universe by studying its smallest elements, the ancient Eastern traditions looked for patterns within the universe as a whole. So when it came to understanding how the human body worked, East and West parted ways once again—but this time *without* reaching a similar understanding.

Much of Western medicine is based upon information obtained from studying cadavers—human beings *without* life or energy. Knowledge of how the body works was sought by *taking it apart*, much as you might disassemble a machine to see how it works. It is easy to see how a lifeless human body could be viewed as a kind of machine. Each organ, vein, artery—everything found within the body—had a clear physical presence, and was assigned its own specific part to play. Therefore, as in a machine, each part could theoretically be taken out and replaced—seemingly without affecting the rest of the system. In fact, organ transplants are well on their way to becoming a routine practice in Western medicine. But this analogy was then extended so that Western medicine came to view *living* human beings as machines as well.

The "life force," the energy that distinguished the corpse from a living person, was something unknowable that simply made this "human machine" run—or cease to run. The nature of our energy was dismissed as an unknowable life mystery not only because it could not be seen, but because there were no tools available to *measure* it.

On the other hand, Eastern medicine obtained its information from scientifically observing *living* human beings—that is, human beings with their energy systems still in existence. Each part of the body was defined not by a specific role, but rather by its relationship with the whole person, with both our physical and our "energetic" selves. Each part of the body was viewed not in terms of how it functioned on its own, but rather in terms of how it functioned in relationship to the entire system. For example, a diseased kidney would not be taken out or replaced. Instead, the *whole system* would be treated. The cause of the disease was not seen as the kidney itself. The diseased kidney was just a sign that there was an energy imbalance in the entire system that had to be corrected. By looking at the body in this holistic way, Eastern practitioners discovered a highly organized system of energy channels or pathways, another circulatory system apart from the cardiovascular and nervous systems. This system could not be seen directly by the human eye, but was proven to be the body's integral means of maintaining its overall well-being.

There is a common misconception in the West that the energy system and the nervous system are actually the same thing. This is not so. The two systems do run in similar patterns throughout 70 percent of the body, sometimes intersecting, sometimes running parallel at different levels. The main reason for this is that the nervous system almost encompasses the entire body, so it is practically impossible to avoid. Still, the energy system is a completely different system, and 30 percent of the time it runs in completely different patterns. But like everything else in the universe and in our bodies, our energy and nervous systems are distinct, yet intimately connected. (We will take an in-depth look at this network of energy channels in the next chapter.)

Because Western medicine is based on studying bodies that have lost their energy systems through death, it has resisted accepting the very existence, much less importance, of the body's energy system. This resistance continues, even though many Western scientists have begun to prove otherwise.

In the 1930s, Dr. Harold Burr of Yale University began experimenting with a voltameter to measure the electrical currents he believed existed within living people as well as within animals and plants. He found similar "electrodynamic force fields" in all three. Two contemporary scientists, Bjorn Nordenstrom, a Swedish radiologist, and Robert Becker, an American orthopedic surgeon, reached similar findings in their research. In his renowned book, *The Body Electric,* * Dr. Becker describes his fascination with tissue regeneration, the process whereby living organisms will grow back duplicates of parts that have been severed. While we take this natural process for granted when it comes to plants, it also occurs more often than you are probably aware of in both animals and people. For example, both a salamander's tail and the fingertip of a small child will automatically replace themselves if severed. Dr. Becker explains this mysterious process by concluding there exists "unifying bioelectric properties" of all living beings.

---

* See Robert O. Becker, M.D., and Gary Selden, *The Body Electric: Electromagnetism and the Foundation of Life* (New York: William Morrow, 1985).

In 1979, after thirty years of research, Dr. Nordenstrom compiled his findings in a book called *Biologically Closed Electrical Circuits: Clinical, Experimental, and Theoretical Evidence for an Additional Circulatory System*. He writes that he found "a complex electrical system" within the human body that regulates organ activity and maintains health. Dr. Nordenstrom became famous for treating tumors with special electrical probes, and discussed his findings at an acupuncturists convention I attended in San Francisco a few years ago. He found he could not only shrink tumors with these electrical probes, but also *increase* their size by reversing the polarity. But what was most amazing to those of us listening to him was that he did not know *why* this occurred. Later on I discussed this with one of my acupuncturist colleagues and we both agreed that although Dr. Nordenstrom would most likely be credited with the discovery of the human energy system in Western science, he was actually the only person, in that roomful of acupuncturists, to not understand his own findings. Eastern medicine has been using this "sedation or tonification" acupuncture technique to manipulate energy for thousands of years. It basically depletes the energy that makes the tumor grow. Again, Western science had stumbled upon ancient healing techniques without realizing it.

Further "visible" evidence of life energy, sufficient to satisfy even the most hardened skeptic, was found through Kirlian photography, a sophisticated photographic technique developed by two Russian scientists, the husband and wife team Semyon and

Valentina Kirlian. They, too, discovered evidence of similar "electromagnetic" fields, and then developed the pictures to prove it. The Kirlians found these energy fields actually extend beyond the physical forms of all living organisms to create what many people describe as "auras." Using their photographic technology, scientists have further discovered that these auras actually reflect the state of health of the organism. A healthy plant's aura was found to be larger and brighter than a dying plant's. The same phenomenon was found in animals and people. Furthermore, human emotions were also found to affect auras. A relaxed, happy person emits a larger, brighter and different colored aura than a tense, unhappy person.

Why have the findings of Western scientists, as well as dozens of others, been virtually ignored by the general Western scientific community? First, Western science has had a relatively brief period of exposure to this system. Eastern scientists and doctors have had about a ten thousand-year head start on the West in the study of energetics. Once they, too, did not believe things existed beyond what the human eye could see. But through trial and error, over thousands of years, they discovered this whole other critical aspect of human existence. So why didn't Western science, as a whole, simply *accept* these findings and build on them, instead of practically starting from scratch? This is a much more difficult question to answer, as it involves the massive political and social changes that continue to affect our global community. It also has to do with some very powerful human emotions, including fear and competitiveness. But to really understand why Western science still resists the existence of an organized energy system within the human body, you have to look at the thought processes dominating today's Western culture.

Research has discovered that specific human thought processes are controlled by the left and right hemispheres of the brain (see table 1).

TABLE I

Left Brain	Right Brain
Time	Space
Rationality	Intuition
Linear Thought	Circular Thought
Deductive Reasoning	Inductive Reasoning
Mathematics	Geometry
Technology	Creativity

Ideally, the two sides of the brain should work in harmony, like *yin* and *yang*. But Western science has apparently resulted from more left-brain than right-brain thought processes. And Western science dominates Western culture. That is, as a culture, we have a tendency to overanalyze ourselves to the point of irrational behavior. We have allowed "logic" to separate us from the universe—to make us see it as something "other" than ourselves. For example, until very recently, we failed to understand our relationship to the environment. In our futile quest to control nature, we have upset the natural balance of our environment and simultaneously upset our own natural balance, our own health. On the other hand, the ancient Eastern traditions were created with more emphasis on right-brain thinking. Man is viewed through his relationship to the universe. (Where a "right-brain" person looks for similarities and associations a "left-brain" person looks for differences.) For Westerners, initial study of tai chi chuan, yoga, and other Eastern holistic health practices will begin to increase right-brain thinking by developing awareness of the "inner self." But what tai chi chuan and yoga ultimately do in advanced study is fuse and balance left- and right-brain processes, something the entire world can benefit from. Just as the East could benefit from more left-brain medical technology, the West could benefit from more Eastern right-brain health practices. In fact, Eastern and Western science need to come together, to balance the thinking processes behind both systems. Both have been spending too much time looking at only half the picture.

Because of Western science's limitations, it is difficult to even discuss energetics using the English language. Language reflects what is valued and understood within a culture. The English language gives us few terms with which to understand the very complicated subject of energy, and none at all to describe the mysterious life force itself. Snow is such an important part of the Eskimo culture that they have many words for it, each term emphasizing a slightly different aspect of it. For example, one word may mean melting snow, another icy snow, and so on. In fact, it may mean the difference between life and death for an Eskimo to be able to understand and decipher the exact kind of snow around him.

The same holds true for Eastern cultures when it comes to energy. The Chinese have hundreds of words for the different types of energy in the body alone. In our Western culture we can only describe someone as "having a lot of energy" when we see them move around in an active manner. When we are tired we say we "have no energy" or feel "drained." We associate our own energy with *physical activity.* We measure it by how much we got done, how many games of tennis we played, and so on. We cannot "realize" our energy unless we see someone or something *move.*

To understand where Western science, as well as much of the rest of the world, currently stands in terms of energetics, imagine yourself trying to show someone from the 1950s how the remote control device you use to change television stations works. You push a button and, "like magic," the channel changes! There are no wires, no *visible* means of changing the channel. But if someone stands between the remote control and the television, nothing happens. Your time-traveler from the fifties would think it was unreal, some kind of trick. (Think of all the forms of energy *we* have seen evidence of, and still do not understand or believe in, such as telekinesis, mental telepathy, and psychic healing.)

Western science created that remote control device, and recognizes the existence of the energy behind the invisible beam it emits. We may not fully understand *how* it works, but we all agree that it does indeed work. Eastern healing traditions have proven that similar invisible "beams" of energy exist with us. They, too, do not fully understand how it works, but fully accept that it does. This book will help you begin to realize this energy as it exists within yourself. Even though you live in a culture dominated by left-brain "seeing is believing" thought processes, you can realize it—you can learn to feel, understand, and control the energy system that exists within you.

Now that you believe (hopefully) in the existence of your own energy system, let's take a look at its three primary aspects. We will call the first one your prenatal or *genetic energy*. This energy forms the basic blueprint of your life and your physical characteristics, from the color of your hair to the shape of your body, and, most likely, determines your life span. We can describe it as the energy contained within the sperm and egg that predated your existence. It is the energy that created the DNA within your every cell. It contains instructions, basically providing an overall plan for your future (similar to the energy described as *purusha* in the ancient Indian tradition).

The second type of energy you have is called your *core energy* (or *prakrita*). This is the energy acquired at conception that worked to form your being. It is the result of the combination of your two prenatal energies. It is the force that carried out the plans, fulfilled the vision of your design.

These two basic energies—genetic energy and core energy—are life forces over which you have no control: They are energies inherited from your ancestors. But there is a third type of energy, called *acquired energy*, over which you have total control. This is the energy you use to run your system. *Acquired energy is the type of energy we are referring to throughout this book.* You may not be able to change your inherited physical traits but, as you will see in later chapters, you can use and control the energies you draw upon throughout your life to help determine the *quality* of your life, and even possibly the length of it.

For example, say your family has a strong history of diabetes. Not every family member has the disease, but many have developed it. Even though the genetic predisposition may be beyond your control, this does not mean that you will automatically develop the disease. It just means you have a stronger chance of getting this particular illness than someone without this family history would have. By developing this third aspect of your energy you can strengthen your system and lessen your chances of getting it. Or, if you do develop the disease, you can minimize the effects it will have on your health and heighten your chances of overriding it. In fact, developing your acquired energy can actually break the chain of inherited disease and positively affect the energies of your children and future generations.

There is a continuing controversy over the effect that genetics, as opposed to learned behavior, has on overall health. So much of our lifestyle is learned from our parents: the way we eat, sleep, exercise—even the way we look at life. The effect our mental outlook alone has on our health is now being taken much more seriously than it was in the past. In fact, under a new branch of research called psychoneuroimmunology,

Western science is beginning to study the mind's ability to control the body's immune system (See chapter 4). In one of his best-selling books, American surgeon Bernie Siegel describes the tremendous success many of his cancer patients have had in beating their illness through mental imagery.* We still do not know whether genetics or lifestyle plays a larger role in our health. But we *do* know that lifestyle has a great impact on our health, and that we can learn to control the way we live.

There are three specific steps you must take before you can begin to realize your energy. You have already taken the first step by reading this book: You have acknowledged the desire to learn about it. The second step is to take responsibility for your own health. Do not let it overwhelm you. Most people do not understand how the things they use everyday work. From the television remote control to the telephone, it all seems too complicated. In our technological society, we have projected that same sense onto ourselves. Many of us see our bodies as complicated machines that are beyond our control and understanding.

In fact, you alone control your health and well-being, and it is your job to maintain it. Your body knows what it needs. Learn to trust it and listen to it. Your body is constantly adjusting and readjusting to external influences, striving to maintain a natural, balanced state of health. While the temperature around you may quickly drop or rise many degrees, your internal tem-

* See Bernie S. Siegel, M.D., *Love, Medicine & Miracles* (New York: Harper & Row, 1986).

perature will hardly change at all, maintaining its average 98.6 degrees. So you must learn not to impede your body's health-maintaining processes. Doctors may guide you and treatment can certainly save your life, but remember that it is always your body alone that heals itself. A doctor may bandage a wound to ward off infection but the actual healing of that wound, the rejoining of the skin, is all the result of your inner energy at work. There is a saying in medicine, *"Primum nil nocere,"* which means, "First do no harm." In fact, 70 percent of all patients have been to found to recover by themselves. Understand that medical professionals are only catalysts in the process. This book will show you how you alone can augment your natural healing powers. It is, of course, a process that takes time, so continue to go to your doctor for regular examinations. But if you start following the health practices contained in this book you may start leaving your checkups with a clean bill of health instead of a large pile of bills.

Western medicine has achieved so many major advances in the past few decades that Western patients have become somewhat lost in the system, cast as passive participants in their own health care. You must maintain an active role. Due to the small number of doctors and hospitals available to the huge Eastern population, Eastern medicine has always stressed self-reliance—and to a large degree it has worked. Both systems have similar bottom-line survival statistics, with different degrees of success in different areas. I believe we are now moving toward a third, universal system of health care that will combine the best of

Eastern and Western healing practices and increase both systems' survival statistics.

After you take responsibility for your own health and well-being, the third step is to make it a top priority in your life. Nothing is more important. Some people view this as negative, selfish behavior, but nothing could be further from the truth. By putting your own health and well-being first, you are *positively* influencing everyone else around you. You are setting an example for them to follow in their own lives and building an easier, healthier road for your children to follow. Taking care of others begins with taking care of yourself.

Once you take these initial steps you will be ready to realize your own energy. In order to accomplish this you must learn to feel it in yourself. Now it is time to let your right brain operate more freely and to concentrate on your intuition. Intuition is simply a heightened awareness of your own inner energy. We all have it and can develop it. When you let your intuition, or your own inner energy, guide you, you are listening to your body and your feelings without allowing your left brain's "logical" impulses to negate them.

As you begin to realize your energy, you will naturally become more aware of how Western medicine and our culture at large often work against you. People sometimes approach Western doctors with what is considered to be a vague complaint. They just do not feel well in general. If the doctor cannot locate a physical manifestation to back up the complaint—something they can *see*—the patient is dismissed as "healthy"; the complaint is seen to exist "only in his head." From an energetics viewpoint, if you *feel* that something is wrong, then something *is* wrong. As you develop your inner energy, you will stop questioning your feelings as often as you probably do now. Energetics equates emotional symptoms with physical ones. Mind and body relate to each other like *yin* and *yang*, and cannot be separated.

Disease does not need to manifest itself physically in order to be acknowledged. As recently as about seventy years ago, Western doctors were using sawdust from the floor to dress wounds. Harmful microorganisms could not be seen, so they were not thought to exist. The doctors did not associate this routine practice with the resulting infections for many years.

Western medicine has been very popular because it seems to offer so many shortcuts to health. Realize that, although there is always more for everyone to learn, Western medicine in particular is still a relatively new science, and the long-term effects of other routine practices, as well as chemically-based pills, have yet to be seen. Eastern healing techniques, on the other hand, have been around for thousands of years. The long-term results are in. The road to health is a long one. There are no shortcuts.

People frequently say, "Listen to your feelings," or, "Follow your heart," while simultaneously criticizing each other for being "too sensitive." Because Western culture often associates sensitivity with weakness, many of us have learned to downplay or deny our feelings. Every once in a while you may have had a "feeling" that something was going to happen and it did. Or perhaps you were once offered a job that seemed like a wonderful opportunity; there was no "reason" to decline, but a feeling told you not to take it and you turned it down. Later you saw that you made the right decision. All these feelings are just your body and your being trying to tell you what it needs to stay healthy and happy. Developing your sensitivity to your own feelings (while maintaining a balanced left-brain ability to discern them), leads to strength, not weakness.

So all you need to do to realize your energy is to get in touch with it. Sound easy? In some ways it is, but with all the distractions of today's increasingly fast-paced, complex world, it is also the hardest thing you will ever accomplish. But once you realize your own inner energy and learn to let it guide you, it will change your life forever. You can learn to enjoy greater health than you ever thought possible and maintain a feeling of well-being no matter what stresses are working against you in your life. It is free, and at your disposal twenty-four-hours-a-day, seven-days-a-week. And just like "the force" in the movie *Star Wars*, it has always been with you.

Realizing your energy begins with developing your sensitivity to it. While it is always with you, its presence within your life is very subtle and elusive. Dr. John Upledger is an osteopathic surgeon in Florida who discovered the power of energetic healing in the 1960s in a desperate attempt to help patients who were not responding to any kind of Western treatment. Using hypodermic needles to stimulate acupuncture or energy points (discussed in chapter 3) on these patients' bodies, he saw amazing results. Now one of the leading exponents of the cranial sacral technique, an innovative approach to energetic healing, Dr. Upledger uses the following visualization to help people understand the elusive nature of their own energy:

> Close your eyes and picture yourself standing perfectly still in the middle of a forest. In your hand you are holding a carrot. A timid deer comes up to you and stands two feet away. The deer represents your energy. In order to contact it you hold the carrot out to it. If you move or take the tiniest step forward it will run away. You extend your arm toward the deer. Although you are standing perfectly still, you are actively concentrating on the carrot in your hand, trying to attract the deer. By concentrating, you are engaging your own energy. The deer slowly moves toward you and begins to eat the carrot in your hand while you continue to remain perfectly still. You are now in perfect control and are perfectly relaxed *at the same time.* This is how it feels to contact your energy.

I use this and a second analogy, which follows, to help my patients begin to visualize engaging their energy systems:

> This time close your eyes and picture yourself standing in a swimming pool. The water is as high as your chest. A piece of tissue paper floats on the surface before you. This time the tissue paper represents your energy. You now not only want to make contact with it, you also want to move it slightly. You extend your hand in the water as if to touch it from underneath. You move as close as possible to it *without physically touching it.*

You are so close you are touching it without touching it. That is, you are touching its "aura," the energy being emitted from it. You feel the energy with the palm of your hand. Concentrating, you move the tissue paper slowly along the surface.

You have now visualized both contacting and controlling your energy. (We will be discussing the specific sensations you can expect to feel when in touch with your energy, including warmth and static electricity, in later chapters.)

Now you can begin to understand the subtle and elusive nature of your energy. Contacting it requires complete stillness or passivity and, concurrently, complete concentration and activity. In other words, you must achieve a perfect *yin/yang* balance. Both analogies also illustrate the extremely delicate action required to contact your energy. If you move too slowly or not enough you won't reach it. If you move too quickly or reach out too far, you'll lose it. The high level of sensitivity it requires is the reason most people miss it.

Next you may need to redefine some visual images you associate with the idea of "energy." When you visualize "energy" or "power," images of explosions, fast cars, or a boxer knocking out his opponent may come to mind. While the energy behind these images is essentially the same as that within your body, your energy is a *delicate* force. In fact, the more delicate and controlled the movement, the more powerful the effect. Think of your energy as if it were a frisbee. Flinging it with all your strength will not send it anywhere near the distance of a sharp, concentrated flick of the wrist.

It may be difficult to understand the power of subtlety, the activity within stillness. But understanding these concepts is an important part of understanding energetics. As we will see in chapter 6, Eastern health practices like tai chi chuan, yoga, and the martial arts are all based on these energetic concepts. They require a sense of stillness and complete concentration so you can begin working with your body to help it reach the balance it is constantly striving for. The focused mental concentration associated with these practices also works to clear the mind of all thoughts, allowing the energy to circulate more freely.

Your energy defies logic, and realizing it is like developing what is known as the "sixth" sense—your intuition and perceptive abilities. The process of getting in touch with this "extra" sense begins with becoming more aware of the five that precede it.

The most powerful sense, energetically speaking, is the sense of smell. The aroma of your favorite meal cooking, the scent of a particular perfume, the smell of smoke from a fire, can all trigger very powerful reactions. These aromas can instantly translate into emotions stored in your memory—which are simply other energy manifestations (see chapter 4). The scent of your favorite meal may remind you of the home you grew up in. Time becomes meaningless as you reexperience sensations first felt years before. Scent-generated memories help you realize the power of your own energy.

Now concentrate on touching things around you.

Pick up a glass. Feel how cold it is. Pick up a wool blanket. Feel how warm it is. Why do some things feel cold and others warm when both exist at "room temperature?" Some things can more easily retain heat, a form of energy, than others. (The same holds true for people. Some of us are just naturally warmer than others.) Now hold the glass in your hands and feel it get warmer. You are transferring your energy to it; your energy is interacting with the glass's energy. Think about energy as you touch wood, metal, a piece of silk. Concentrate on realizing the different energies contained in everything around you.

Next focus on the energy contained in different sounds. Think about how you interact with them. A sudden bang will "hurt" your ears. Soft music may relax you. All these energies, simply manifested as different sounds, are again, reacting with your own energy. It is no accident that as people get older, their taste in music generally changes from loud rock 'n' roll to softer classical music. Why does the same music that made us feel like dancing all night in our teens give us a headache in our fifties? Looking at it from an energetic viewpoint, as we age and we feel our inner energy start to diminish, we generally become more sensitive and appreciative of it and its subtle, complex nature. We then, in turn, apply these same feelings to the world around us. We suddenly appreciate the subtle complexities of a Mozart sonata, the same piece of music we may have found boring in our youth.

The same may be said for the sense of taste. The pizza and hot dogs that thrilled us as children are now replaced by delicate sauces subtly seasoned by master chefs. Again, the food has not changed, we have. As we mature, life actually allows us to become more fully aware of the many different aspects of our own inner energy, thus giving us the ability to appreciate the full spectrum of ingredients in a delicately flavored sauce.

The last of our five senses, sight, also triggers powerful energetic reactions in a variety of ways, usually by reinforcing the other four. Although all five senses work together to keep us in touch with the energies around us, some of us will have developed one sense more than another. One person will be able to smell the difference between two perfumes that seem exactly the same to someone else. Another person will be able to pick out an oboe playing in a classical piece that another person cannot hear at all. Accordingly, when the balance of our five senses is upset, the remaining senses will compensate, striving to maintain the body's natural overall balance. For example, a blind person's hearing abilities will generally become augmented as the body compensates for the loss of sight. And your sixth sense, your powers of intuition, works with all your other senses to oversee all of your being. It serves to maintain both your physical and mental health. As you read the next few chapters, continue to develop your awareness of your energy so you will be ready to learn how to increase and control it through the diet, lifestyle, and exercise guidelines in chapters 5 and 6.

As you become more aware of how you use your senses to contact the energies around you, you can also start to concentrate on the energies of other people.

The more in touch you are with the energies around you, the more you will be in touch with the energy within yourself, and vice versa. There is continual interaction between the energies of individuals, which feeds back into the internal energy system of each person. Again, look at our use of language: Someone may make you feel better by "just being there"; when we say goodbye we say "keep in touch." Think about how other people affect your energy. Young children have enormous amounts of energy. Spending time with them usually begins as an invigorating experience and often ends up as an exhausting one. What about the expression "misery loves company?" Frequently people who are depressed lack energy. After a few hours, you feel depressed and exhausted just being around them. Yet with other people who are vibrant and active, you feel you could spend days talking to them. These people have balanced energy. Since our energies interact, people who lack energy can literally "drain" others as they subconsciously try to balance out their own systems, whereas healthier people with balanced internal energy can peacefully coexist with other people. We will take a closer look at this phenomenon later, when we discuss the relationship between your emotions and your energy.

While this book is designed to familiarize you with just the basic principles behind energetic healing, following the guidelines presented here can lead to extraordinary results. When you learn to concentrate your energy you are learning to develop your willpower. In advanced stages, you will be able to concentrate your energy at will. This is what professional athletes call "zoning" and what artists refer to as "divine inspiration," and is closely related to the level of energy called "*mahat*" in the Indian tradition (see figure 2 in the previous chapter).

When in this "higher zone," the human brain operates like a computer, processing information at superhuman speeds. At this level tennis players serve ace after ace, world-class chess players plot moves hours before they make them, concert pianists watch their hands effortlessly play the most difficult composition. Their energy is so concentrated that they can actually detach themselves from the activity; they can almost literally move their physical selves out of the way. The human body suddenly becomes a very controlled, efficient system.

Jay Leno, the popular comedian, discussed "zoning" in a recent interview with *Playboy* magazine.* "When I do two two-hour shows, which is fairly often," Leno said, "I get into the rhythm of the thing and I fall asleep on stage. I just plain go out for about forty minutes and then come back in again and drift in and out . . . [O]ther comics know what I'm talking about. You get on a roll with the audience. A friend of mine put one of those pulse things on me and boy, my pulse drops *waaay* down when I'm on stage." That is exactly what happens in "zoning." At this level of consciousness, your energy is so concentrated that your heartbeat slows down even while you are in full control of all your functions. You can actually release the

* Dick Lochte, "Playboy Interview: Jay Leno," *Playboy* (December 1990).

amount of adrenaline you need when you need it. When you reach this level of concentration, you control your life, it does not control you. It takes a lot of time, discipline, and self-motivation to reach this level of consciousness—but anyone can do it.

As a former professional martial artist, I have had many experiences with "zoning." One of the most memorable occurred several years ago while I was attending a formal banquet in Hong Kong honoring a great kung fu master on his eightieth birthday. I stood next to him as a large crowd of accomplished martial artists came to pay their respects. It was considered a very special honor to greet him at his table.

Suddenly a young street punk, obviously drunk, appeared out of nowhere and began shouting insults at the master. He then challenged the master to a fight. This disrespectful behavior was completely unheard of, something no one in his right mind would ever do. "You're just a fake," the street kid said to the master as we all stared in disbelief. Now, I had previously seen this eighty-year-old man floor young men twice this kid's size with one simple palm strike. Although the master said nothing and showed absolutely no outward sign, I knew there was going to be trouble.

There was no time to plan strategy, only time to act. As I worked my way through the crowd, I focused my entire concentration on this offensive intruder. He saw me approaching and immediately attacked with a vicious swinging punch. By this time I had reached the "zoning" level of concentration. I seemed to know what this kid was going to do before he did it. It was as if I had choreographed the scene long ago. I was completely relaxed yet fully concentrated as I used simple defensive blocks to divert his blows. It worked like magic. I almost could not believe that he was doing everything exactly as I had imagined it, as if he were doing what I told him to do.

The whole fight probably lasted only five or six seconds but, to me, it seemed to progress in slow-motion. At this high level of concentration, you can actually go out of phase with the universal energy (that is, have an out of body experience) and get into a position where you objectively observe the situation. It is the feeling of watching yourself perform an activity. Described by many people as "out-of-body experiences," these are very real phenomena.

Most people in the room only saw a drunken man bump into me, fall backward, and then get jumped on by a crowd of angry martial artists. But while many people there felt they had defended the master, only one person knew what had actually happened—the kung fu master himself, who silently nodded to me from across the room. (The offender was then dragged before him on his knees to beg forgiveness, and later forced to leave Hong Kong forever.)

This chapter's initial question was, "What does energetics have to do with me?" You can now see that the answer is *everything*. When it comes to your overall well-being, your energy is your greatest resource. When you are in touch with it, you are in touch with your own power. It is so subtle that it is difficult to perceive. You must travel within yourself to find it. But once you do find it, you will be aware of it always. This book will help you get there, but you alone will know when you have arrived. Your energy is the key to your own health and happiness. Think of it as a wave that has its own rhythm. Let it take you where you want to go, and leave your left-brain thinking at the door.

Chapter Three

HOW ENERGY WORKS
IN YOUR BODY

You ALREADY know much more about how energy works in your body than you probably realize. Every time you instinctively rub a banged knee or try to get warm by rubbing your palms together, you are activating your body's energy system. The pain you felt after banging your knee was your brain alerting you to an energy blockage in your body. The brain is extremely sensitive to any change or disruption of energy flow. Rubbing the knee released the blocked energy and so eased the pain. Again, although all are distinct systems unto themselves, the brain, nervous system and energy system are all intimately related and inseparable. Banging your knee disrupted the flow of energy within the nerves of that knee. By allowing you to feel pain, your brain told you this had happened. Touch the centers of the palms of your hands. Even if your hands are chronically cold you will feel two warm spots there. There are two important energy centers or points. By simply rubbing your palms together you are stimulating these points and sending energy in the form of warmth throughout your body.

Before you learn the specifics behind how energy circulates in your body, you need to understand more about the energy itself. The energy that flows within our bodies is more than electricity or the result of chemical reactions. It has many different aspects that work together as a mysterious life force. Attempts to "dissect" our energy have raised more questions than answers. Each aspect can only be understood in terms of how it works together with the others. But one of the most mysterious and fascinating aspects of our "human" energy is that it can carry *information* in the form of specific messages to other parts of our being. Just as the DNA within our every cell contains the genetic "plans" for our physical beings—and possibly our psychological beings as well—our *qi*, or life energy, also contains this potential. The important difference is that we can learn to control this life energy—to "program" it ourselves. As you will see in the next chapter, we can use our intelligence to direct our energy, to send it where we want it to go; furthermore, we can "tell" it what we want it to do. The problem is that we are just beginning to learn how to do this. Science has just begun to accept this truth, and to study the many unexplained phenomena like ESP (extra sensory perception) that have been ignored or dismissed as magic or coincidence. Every day we are learning more about our own power, our own energy, and about how to develop it and use it. Yet, while we are just beginning to study the universal truths behind the energy that flows within us, and learn more about its mysterious and complex nature, we already understand a lot about *how* it flows, at least in terms of patterns and directions.

Governed by *yin* and *yang*, sometimes described as positive and negative charges, our energy flows along very specific but invisible channels or pathways throughout our bodies. This complex network forms a veritable energy "road map." But these "lines of energy" are actually just the centers of many three-dimensional fields that together comprise our internal energy system and our external aura, much like the energy fields surrounding magnets.

Pain or illness results when the flow of energy becomes blocked or unbalanced in some way, because this disharmony then upsets the balance of the body's entire energy system. There are many different sub-systems at work within our complex energy system. Just as our main arteries break off into a myriad of tiny blood vessels that move blood throughout the body, so do our main energy channels break down into smaller channels in order to supply us with the energy we need and carry messages to the brain and throughout the entire body. Although some energetic healing techniques engage the entire system, many only need to work with the body's twelve primary channels and two governing vessels (channels that oversee all others) to create complete balance and health.

Each of the twelve primary channels corresponds to one of the body's twelve primary energetic organs. In energetic medicine, an organ, too, is actually an energy system that can only be understood in its relationship to the body's entire energy system. For example, the lung refers to the energy that flows through the lung channel to regulate the lungs, as well as through the physical organ itself. Furthermore, it is interesting to note that although each physical organ has specific corresponding energy fields, the energy fields precede the physical structures. The energy came first. Just as the size of tumors can be increased or decreased by manipulating energy flow, so too can the physical development of any internal organ be prevented by blocking the associated flow of energy. Our physical structures do not first exist and then "radiate" energy; our energy determines our physical structure.

It is necessary, first, to have a general overview of how each of the twelve primary channels and two governing vessels work. While every channel in our bodies exists in perfect bilateral symmetry, each one functions and runs differently. Although depth cannot be depicted in the following illustrations, some energy channels originate internally and end on the surface of the body, others do the exact opposite—and there are many variations in between. The arrows indicate the proper direction of energy flow. A detailed description of the exact nature of even one channel is beyond the scope of this book. The following descriptions are only meant to provide you with a basic introduction to your energy system. Included are lists of a few ailments that could possibly result from an improper flow of energy within each specific channel.

1. Lung Channel.

The lung channel begins near the navel. The energy first moves downward to the large intestine and then upward through the lungs. The channel surfaces near the collarbones before splitting into two and moving down each arm to finally end at the tip of each thumb.

The lung channel regulates the entire energy system of the body. Besides meaning "energy," *qi* and *prana* also directly translate as "air." Obviously, acquiring oxygen is the primary way we acquire energy throughout our lives. From the moment of conception, it is our most immediate need for survival, so it makes sense that this first energy channel works to regulate all others. And that is why learning proper breathing techniques is so important in maintaining your overall energy system, and why it is such an important part of tai chi chuan, yoga, and any kind of exercise. An energy blockage in the lung channel would, like all other energy blockages, upset the overall balance of the body's entire energy system. Disharmony here is often experienced as coughing, asthma, allergies, skin problems, bronchitis, and fatigue.

Lu. 1

Zhongjiao

Lu. 7

Lu. 11

The unbroken line shows the channel.
The broken line shows the internal connections of the channel.

The Lung Channel

2. Large Intestine Channel.

This channel begins at the tip of each index finger and runs up to the shoulders. Here it splits into two branches on each side; one heads down through the lungs to the large intestine, the other moves along the skin's surface and ends on the opposite side of the nose. The energy contained in this system is that which supports the body's ability to remove waste. Disharmony in the energy within the large intestine channel could result in a distended abdomen, constipation, or diarrhea.

FIGURE 4

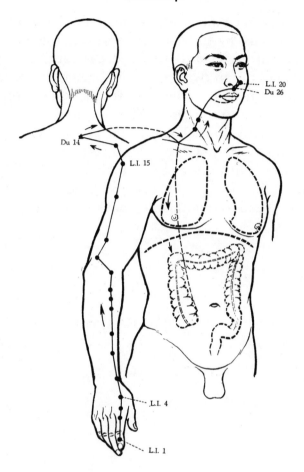

The Large Intestine Channel

3. Stomach Channel.

The stomach channel begins where the large intestine channel ends, by the nose. It moves first down to the jaw, then up each side of the head. Back at the jaw point it branches out in two directions. One branch heads for the stomach and spleen, the second runs along the skin's surface to the groin. The two branches then re-join internally on each side of the groin, then separate again and move down each leg, ending at second toes. The energy within the stomach channel regulates the body's ability to take in food and fluids. Disharmony here may lead to mouth sores, nausea, or vomiting.

FIGURE 5

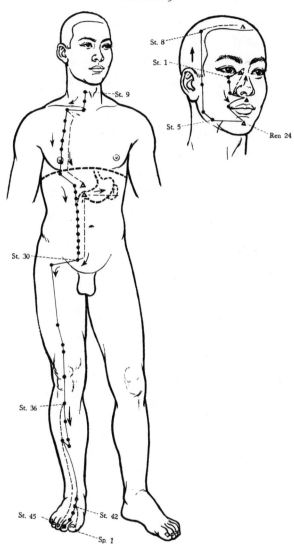

St. 8

St. 1

St. 9

St. 5

Ren 24

St. 30

St. 36

St. 45

St. 42

Sp. 1

The Stomach Channel

4. Spleen Channel.

The spleen channel begins at each big toe and moves up the legs and through the body cavity to the spleen. The energy then moves up the throat, ending at the base of the tongue. The energy from this channel system is primarily responsible for transforming food into energy, but it also regulates the maintenance of the body's blood. Disharmony within this energy channel could result in poor appetite, anemia, menstrual problems, chronic hepatitis, or fatigue.

FIGURE 6

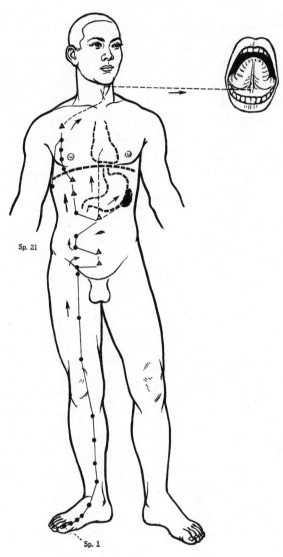

Sp. 21

Sp. 1

The Spleen Channel

5. Heart Channel.

Three branches of this channel originate on each side of the body in the heart. One of the branches on each side moves downward to the small intestine, the second runs upward to the eye, and the third runs across the chest and down the inside of the arm, terminating at the inside tip of the little finger. The energy that circulates in the heart channel is said to rule the head and house the spirit, as well as regulate the body's blood vessels. An unbalanced flow of energy here may lead to heart palpitations or insomnia.

FIGURE 7

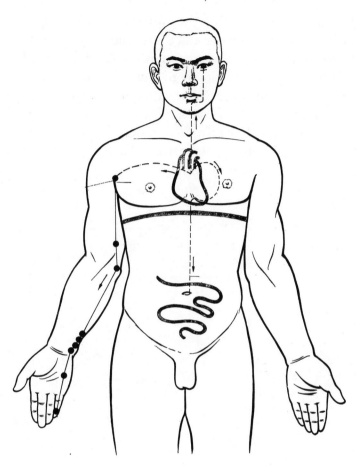

The Heart Channel

6. Small Intestine Channel.

This channel begins at the outside tip of each little finger, runs up the arms and then around the shoulders to the center of the back. Here it resplits into two branches; one moves down to the small intestine, the second moves up to the cheek and ends within the ear. This energy channel functions to draw out the energy contained in food, leaving the remaining matter to be eliminated as waste. Disharmony here may result in vomiting or abdominal pain.

FIGURE 8

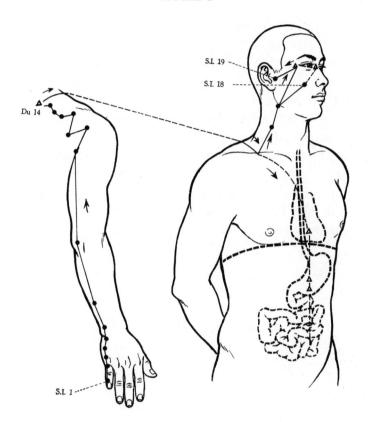

The Small Intestine Channel

7. *Bladder Channel.*

Beginning at the inner side of each eye, the bladder channel first moves up to the top of the head. It then runs along the back of the head and separates into two channels on each side of the back of the neck. One branch then moves internally, parallel to the spine, down to the bladder. The second, outer branch moves downward adjacent to the spinal cord. The two branches then rejoin behind each knee and end at the tip of each small toe. This channel works to receive and excrete urine (fluid waste). An unbalanced flow of energy in the bladder channel could result in burning sensations when urinating or incontinence.

FIGURE 9

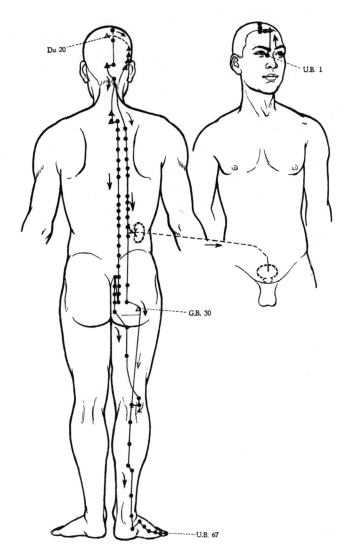

The Bladder Channel

8. Kidney Channel.

The kidney channel begins under each big toe and moves up each inner leg, eventually connecting with the kidney. From there it moves upward, ending near the collarbone. A second branch also begins in the kidney and moves upward on each side, ending at the base of the tongue. The body's reproductive energy is stored in the kidney channel, which also oversees the maintenance of the body's bones. Problems arising from an improper flow of energy in this channel can result in backache, chronic ear problems, or chronic asthma.

FIGURE 10

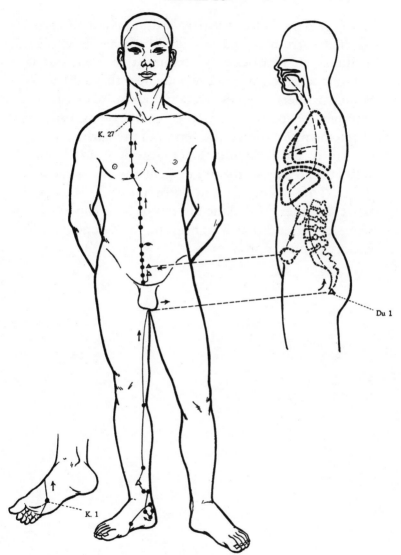

K. 27

Du 1

K. 1

The Kidney Channel

9. Pericardium Channel.

In Western medicine, the pericardium is a membranous sac that surrounds and protects the heart. In energetic medicine, it is an energy channel that begins as two branches on each side of the body near the heart. As one branch of energy moves straight downward on each side through the body cavity, the second one crosses the chest and moves down the center of each arm, ending at the tip of each middle finger. Another small branch splits off at the palms and ends at the tip of each ring finger. This energy channel protects and oversees the heart channel. Unbalanced energy here can result in stress experienced as a tightening in the chest, or in a variety of breast problems.

FIGURE 11

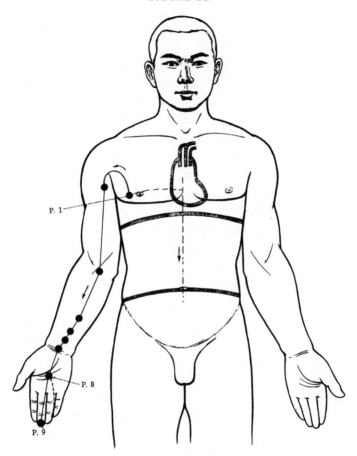

P. 1

P. 8

P. 9

The Pericardium Channel

10. Triple Burner Channel.

As was previously discussed, the way energetic and Western medicine view the internal organs differs greatly. Whereas Western medicine recognizes an organ by its physical structure, energetic medicine defines it by its function. Therefore, energetic medicine recognizes some organs, like the triple burner, that you probably have never heard of before, while organs like the pancreas and adrenal glands are not recognized. But even within energetic medicine the triple burner is difficult to describe and understand. It is a system described as "three burning spaces" in the body, which circulates energy throughout the channel described below, uniting other organs in order to regulate "water" energy (one of the five basic types or phases of energy, as will be explained later) throughout the upper, middle, and lower thirds of the body.

Beginning at the tip of each ring finger, the triple burner channel runs over the back of the hands and then upward toward the shoulders. The energy then moves inward to the chest cavity. From here one inward branch moves downward on each side to unite the middle and lower sections of the body. A second interior branch moves up to each ear and circles the face. This energy channel oversees the body's ability to process water, to retain what it needs and excrete what it cannot use. An improper flow of energy in this channel may be experienced as edema (water retention) or as a stiff neck.

FIGURE 12

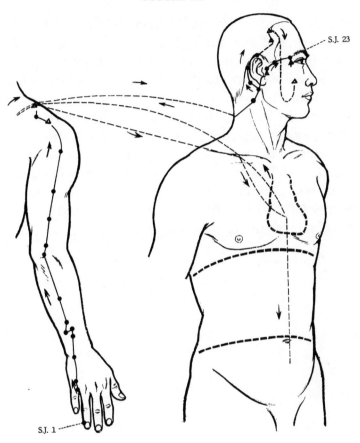

The Triple Burner Channel

11. Gall Bladder Channel.

The gall bladder channel begins with two branches originating at the outer side of each eye. One moves back and forth on the sides of the head, around the ears and then downward to the hip area. The second branch moves internally across each cheek and then downward through the neck to the gall bladder. It then rejoins the other branch and moves down the outside of each leg, then across the top of the feet, ending at the tip of each fourth toe. This energy system works to store and secrete bile, a fluid that aids in transforming food into energy. Disharmony here may be experienced as a bitter taste in one's mouth, nausea, or jaundice.

FIGURE 13

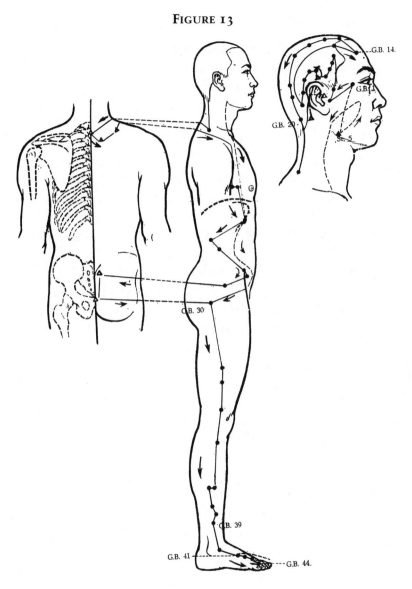

The Gall Bladder Channel

12. Liver Channel.

Like the lung channel, the liver channel also regulates the flow of energy throughout the body. But as the lung channel oversees the intake of "air" energy, the liver channel oversees the maintenance of the body's blood supply.

The liver channel begins on the top of each big toe, moves across the top of the feet and then upward on the inner side of each leg. From here it circles around the external genitalia, then moves up to the liver, eventually connecting with the lung channel in the lungs. The entire circulation of energy begins anew here as the channel moves up the throat to each eye. From here it splits to move down around the lips and across the forehead to the top of the head. An energy imbalance in the liver channel may lead to high blood pressure, dizziness, pre-menstrual syndrome, muscle spasms, or eye problems.

FIGURE 14

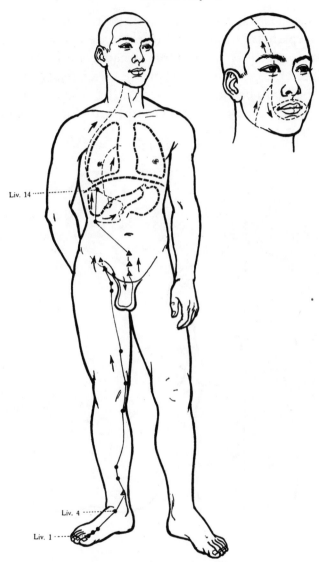

Liv. 14

Liv. 4

Liv. 1

The Liver Channel

13. & 14. Governing Vessel and Conception Vessel.

These two vessels are also sometimes referred to as the last two primary channels. But they are called vessels, and are especially important, because both work to circulate energy through all of the other twelve channels. The main branch of the governing vessel begins at the tip of the coccyx and moves upward along the mid-

FIGURE 15

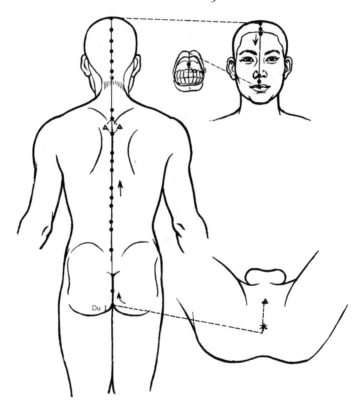

The Governing Vessel

dle of the spinal column. It continues over the top of the head and down the middle of the forehead, and ends below the nose inside the upper gum. The conception vessel begins between the anus and genitalia, then moves upward through the middle body to the lower jaw. Here it moves internally to circle the lips and then branch upward to the eyes.

FIGURE 16

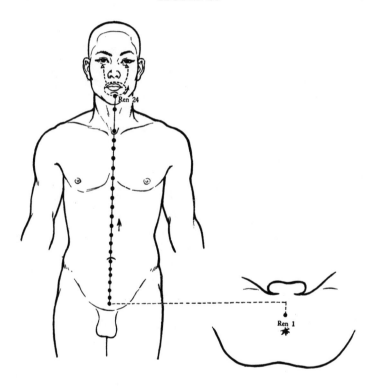

The Conception Vessel

Energy continually circulates through each of these channels, and it also circulates through the body as a whole by intensifying in different channels at different times of the day (see table 2). Therefore, unbalanced energy in any channel may become more unbalanced during certain hours. For example, someone suffering from asthma caused by an energy imbalance in the lung channel would most likely experience an attack or have the most difficulty breathing between three and five in the morning.

Table 2

Energy Channel	Time of Intensified Flow
Gall Bladder	11 P.M. – 1 A.M.
Liver	1 A.M.– 3 A.M.
Lung	3 A.M.– 5 A.M.
Large Intestine	5 A.M.– 7 A.M.
Stomach	7 A.M.– 9 A.M.
Spleen	9 A.M.–11 A.M.
Heart	11 A.M.– 1 P.M.
Small Intestine	1 P.M. – 3 P.M.
Bladder	3 P.M. – 5 P.M.
Kidney	5 P.M. – 7 P.M.
Pericardium	7 P.M. – 9 P.M.
Triple Burner	9 P.M. –11 P.M.

When the energy circulates freely through these channels, and all the other pathways in the body, we are in a state of optimum health and will experience feelings of well-being. But if there is an unbalanced flow of energy in just one of the primary channels or governing vessels, or one of the hundreds of subchannels in our entire system, the balance of our health may be thrown off. Sometimes the problem is easily solved—as by rubbing that banged knee—but oftentimes the problem does not just go away. The energy that flows throughout our bodies may become disrupted in a variety of ways. There may be too much energy flowing in any one channel, or too little in another, or the energy may become blocked or flow in the wrong direction. Any of these problems, left uncorrected over a long period of time, can lead to a serious illness.

If the energy in your body does become unbalanced, then what do you do? You now have a basic understanding of how energy flows throughout your body, but how can you use this information? With someone suffering from chronic asthma, is their energy imbalance in the lung channel or the kidney channel? And what caused the energy to stop flowing properly in the first place? The answer to all of these questions lies within what is called a *pattern of disharmony.*

Just as universal truths lie within the patterns of the universe, so does the truth behind the cause of an illness lie within ourselves. Like a detective solving a mysterious crime, the energetic therapist (whether you or a professional) must find *recurrent themes* within the symptoms and signs of disharmony. Each theme is another clue that will lead to the source of the energy imbalance. Therefore, in order to find this pattern and correct it, as much information as possible must first be gathered. (In this chapter we are limiting ourselves to patterns within the body. In the next chapter we will discuss locating patterns within the mind as well.)

Although much depends upon the current state of

your health, it is still often both necessary and wise to consult a professional energetic therapist—a qualified doctor of Oriental medicine with an O.M.D. degree or any trained energetic therapist with proper credentials (see appendix for a list of referral sources). The next few chapters will show you how you yourself can balance your own energy, but these skills take time to learn and develop. An energetic therapist can speed up the healing process and the learning process behind regulating your own energy balance.

This process begins with the enormous task of gathering the necessary information, which is done in three stages. The first stage is identifying your initial symptom(s)—the problem that alerted you to the existence of your energy imbalance. After you describe your problem to the therapist, he or she will begin to look for the next source of information—*signs* of illness. You may exhibit a symptom you are not even aware of that a professional therapist will recognize as a sign of illness. Signs of disharmony may be found in a stooped posture, a raspy voice, a sense of nervousness, or even brittle nails. This first part of treatment, of collecting information, is a very extensive one. During your first visit to an energetic therapist, expect to spend at least half an hour just talking about your symptoms, feelings, and lifestyle. Every piece of information, no matter how irrelevant it may seem to you, is a part of the puzzle. And just as the puzzle cannot be completed without each piece, the importance of each piece cannot be understood until the puzzle is completed.

The second stage of information gathering involves a thorough examination of your tongue. Most Western doctors look at the tongue very quickly, but an energetic therapist will study it closely because its appearance answers many basic questions. Signs of disharmony may lie in the color of the tongue, the size and shape of it, or just in the color and thickness of its coating. Ridges around the tongue point to an excess of water in the body. A red-tipped tongue may indicate blocked energy in the heart channel.

After talking to you and checking your tongue, the therapist will begin the third stage of information gathering: taking your pulse—or, actually, your *pulses.* As opposed to the "single" pulse used by Western medicine to monitor the cardiovascular system, energetic medicine recognizes twelve pulses. Each corresponds to one of the primary energy channels. Again, more information is gathered from this practice than that of Western physicians. Placing three fingers on each of the patient's wrists, the therapist takes the pulses on three levels, surface, middle, and deep, checking not only the speed and strength of each pulse, but also the more elusive *qualities* of it—its overall shape, rhythm, and length. It may be difficult to understand what these terms have to do with determining the quality of a pulse, and, in fact, taking a pulse in energetics is very difficult. It requires years of extensive training and a lot of concentration to determine the exact nature of a patient's pulse, but the information is critically important in finding the pattern of disharmony. Each of your twelve pulses gives the therapist specific information about your overall energy, as well as an amazing amount of information concerning some of the primary channels. He or she may report that you have a floating or sinking pulse, or an empty or full one, or one that is slippery or choppy. Don't let these descriptions unnerve you; they are only more pieces of the puzzle the energetic therapist is now beginning to complete.

Once these three relatively simple diagnostic methods are applied, the therapist has a lot of information to work with. But connecting disparate symptoms and signs and weaving them into a pattern of disharmony can be extremely difficult, as you will see in the case studies from my practice in the next chapter. It requires much training, skill, and talent. After all, what do a ruddy complexion, weak nails, and rapid pulse have to do with each other? A skilled energetic therapist would know that they have a lot in common: All three point to an energy imbalance in the liver channel.

But very rarely are all the pieces of the puzzle put together so easily. Energetics recognizes hundreds of patterns of disharmony. In order to find the patient's exact pattern (or patterns), the energetic therapist uses a simple diagnostic model called the *five phases*. Derived from *yin* and *yang* (refer back to figure 1, chapter 1), these five phases of energy, according to the ancient Chinese tradition, are *wood, fire, earth, metal*, and *water*. These terms do not literally refer to the actual matter; instead they are meant to describe five different basic *qualities* of energy, and were originally used in ancient China to classify everything in the universe. Therefore, the energy that flows through the twelve primary channels and two governing vessels has these five basic qualities to it. If all five types of energy are not balanced within each and every channel, the disharmony in any one channel can throw off the delicate balance of the body's entire energy system.

To describe these five qualities or types of energy, and to help you identify them within yourself, each must be associated with a distinct set of feelings or emotions. Understood in this way, they create a simple diagnostic model and give the energetic therapist a classification system that facilitates the task of organizing disparate signs and symptoms into a cohesive, understandable pattern of disharmony.

Like *yin* and *yang*, the four seasons, and each stage of our life cycle, each of the five phases cannot be understood alone, but only by its relationship to the others. And, again like *yin* and *yang*, they form a cycle that illustrates how they both control and create each other. The creation cycle shows how each phase gives rise to or creates the next, and the star pattern within the cycle shows how each phase controls and is controlled by the others (see figure 17).

Just as energy could be experienced through the exercises in chapter 1, each of the five phases can be experienced by imagining them and/or actually touching the corresponding matter. *Wood* is the quality of energy associated with the season of spring, with the energy behind birth and growth. The feelings associated with wood energy are strength and warmth. *Fire* is the quality of energy associated with the season of summer. It is the energy behind upward growth, the phase that corresponds with childhood. Fire energy feels hot. It is associated with activity, expansion, and all the warm, rising qualities of nature. After fire comes *earth*, the energy of mature adulthood, of late summer when crops are harvested. Earth energy is cool and nurturing. It is the type of energy associated with neutrality and balance. The fourth phase is *metal*, which corresponds to the season

FIGURE 17

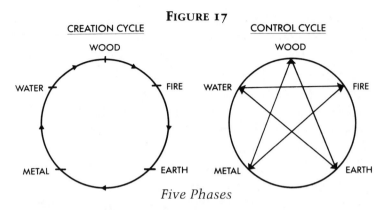

Five Phases

of autumn. This is the energy associated with the beginning of decline and decay, and often with old age. Metal energy is cold, stiff, and hard. The final phase is *water*. As the end of the energy cycle, it represents both death and rebirth. Water is associated with coldness, fluidity, and movement. It is the snow from the tops of mountains that become the streams of spring. Energy is always moving through the cycle of the five phases, just as time moves us through the four annual seasons and the different stages of our lives. Our health lies in the balance of these five phases.

So let's say that in gathering all the patient's information, the energetic therapist connects a ruddy complexion with a red-tipped tongue and then with a rapid pulse. As mentioned before, together they point to an energy imbalance in the heart channel—in this case, excess fire energy. In order to rebalance the energy, the therapist will use a healing technique that either increases water energy, the energy that controls fire energy or else decreases wood energy, the energy that "feeds the fire." This practice can be compared to how you would naturally deal with a thirst acquired by jogging five miles in the hot sun: You would either drink a cold glass of water or you stop jogging—or both.

Just as the five phases of energy must be balanced within every energy channel, so the channels themselves must be balanced with each other. The twelve primary channels are further classified as being associated with one of the five phases. Again, this should not be taken too literally: It just refers to a very subtle overall quality of the energy that flows through each channel (see table 3).

TABLE 3

PHASE:	Wood	Fire	Earth	Metal	Water
SEASON:	Spring	Summer	Late summer	Autumn	Winter
YIN CHANNEL:	Liver	Heart	Spleen	Lungs	Kidney
YANG CHANNEL:	Gall bladder	Small intestine Triple burner Pericardium	Stomach	Large intestine	Bladder
DISHARMONY SEEN IN:	Eyes, Nails	Tongue, Facial complexion	Mouth, Lips	Nose, Skin	Ears, Hair

This chart represents an overly simplified picture of the connections an energetic therapist makes. This is just to help you recognize and understand some of the basic connections behind many intricate patterns of disharmony.

Therefore, in order to keep the energy that maintains your body's natural balance of health moving, the energetic therapist must first be able to identify the exact kind of energy that is not flowing properly, and then balance the energy system by either increasing the controlling quality of energy, decreasing the creative quality of energy, or both. But, as always, it is the patient's energy, and that alone, which accomplishes the actual healing.

My associates and I use many different types of energetic healing techniques at the Q.M. Institute, the energetics clinic I founded in Manhattan. Q.M. stands for *qi kung* manipulation, and is a general term for many different types of therapies that involve energy manipulation. (Qi kung—pronounced "chee goong"—roughly translates to internal energetic activity.) Two of the most effective therapies offered at the institute are acupuncture and Q.M. therapy.

Acupuncture is one of the most widely known and practiced of all the energetic therapeutic techniques. In addition to strengthening the immune system and treating many diseases, it is effective as a natural local anesthetic. Acupuncture is a general term used to describe different methods of balancing the body's energy system by placing hair-thin, stainless steel needles in special sites along the twelve primary energy channels and two governing vessels.

Just as our arteries and nerves are protected by our bodies' muscles, so, too, are our energy channels, so it is often difficult to affect them directly. Acupuncture points are located where the protective layer of muscle is less thick or the energy channel runs close to the surface of the body. They are generally very sensitive points, and are also used as points of attack in martial arts. One acupuncture point that most people are familiar with is what we call our "funny bone," a spot on each elbow where the heart channel runs very close to the surface of the body and intersects the nervous system. A well-placed tap here can cause a severe energy blockage that will momentarily "shut down" the area from the elbow to the tips of the fingers, leaving the entire forearm completely numb.

Acupuncture points are like small energy centers themselves. Different points have different functions; some drain energy, others activate it. Stimulating each of these points with the thin needles works to unblock or balance energy in that channel. The needles, placed at varying depths along the surface of the body, balance the entire interior energy system by in effect interfacing between the "higher energy" of *qi* and our physical body. Using Kirlian photography, researchers have found that changes occur in the brightness of acupuncture points hours, days, or even weeks before an illness manifests itself in the subject. This research not only confirmed the fact that energy imbalances lead to illness, but also showed that energetic therapists can use acupuncture points to detect illnesses in extremely early stages—before any conventional symptoms are apparent—and so reverse the process before any real damage is done.

As you have seen from the illustrations of the primary energy channels, the lung channel circulates between the lung area and the arms. So as treatment for chronic asthma, an energetic therapist may use acupuncture points on the wrist or forearm. Or an energy blockage in the liver channel may call for the stimulation of acupuncture points on the feet. The stimulation of acupuncture or energy points, as we will see in chapter 6, is also one of the basic premises behind many Eastern healing techniques like tai chi chuan and yoga. Certain positions, held over a period of time, are another way of stimulating these energy points and easing the flow of energy throughout the body.

While all acupuncturists work to stimulate the same points along the body's energy channels, there are a variety of ways to go about doing this. To begin with, there are hundreds of different types of needles. And to increase their effectiveness, the needles themselves are often further stimulated with moxibustion (heating in sticks of burning herbs) or a slight electrical charge. But there are a variety of other therapeutic techniques that stimulate acupuncture points as well, including acupressure and shiatsu massage. Different techniques work best for different people but, overall, I have found acupuncture to be the most effective treatment for the greatest variety of illnesses.

Even within the practice of acupuncture, different techniques work best for different people. Although two people may be suffering from a common cold, an energetic therapist may use different combinations of acupuncture points to treat each person. This is because just as no two people's energy systems are alike, no two illnesses are alike—no matter how similar the symptoms may be. Sometimes a therapist may find that the most effective way to treat a patient is by using one of the body's microsystems.

Within the overall energy system exist multiple microsystems, the three primary ones being the ears, feet, and hands. Microsystems are like energetic microcosms of the entire body. An energetic therapist can obtain a lot of information from taking your pulses and looking at your tongue; but working with only these microsystems, all relatively small areas of the body, he or she can actually diagnose and treat illnesses that occur anywhere in the body. Because each of the twelve primary energy channels is connected with these three microsystems either directly or indirectly, points within each area have been found to directly correspond to points throughout the body. The acupuncture points on the ear are even named according to the part of the body with which they are associated, and stimulation of these points will affect that part of the body. It is also interesting to note that the arrangement of the points on the ear often parallels the anatomy of a fetus (see figure 18a and b).

The ear is fast becoming the most widely used microsystem for both diagnosing and treating illness. Many illnesses from hypertension to hepatitis, from the common cold to tonsillitis—can be treated using only points located on the ears. Although other energetic therapies are also used in conjunction with the microsystems, ear acupuncture has become a popular technique used around the world. Just as acupuncture points change in terms of tenderness and electrical charges *before* an illness manifests itself in the body, so do the points on the ear forewarn of disease. Changes in electrical charge, color, and tenderness have been found to correspond to the development of specific diseases throughout the body. Using acupuncture points on the ear alone, an energetic therapist can treat a wide range of illnesses, and even some serious diseases.

The body's twelve primary channels can also be accessed through the feet and hands. Reflexology, a popular therapeutic technique, cures the body of disease by stimulating acupuncture points on the feet. Insomnia, headaches, and back pain are just a few of the

FIGURE 18A & B

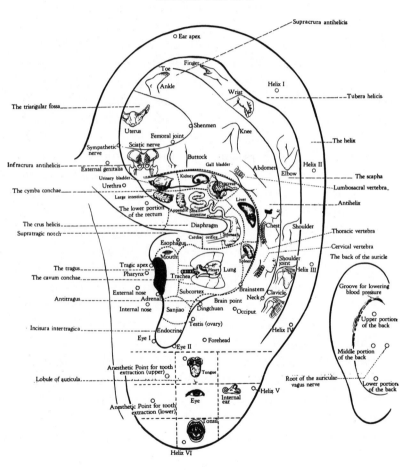

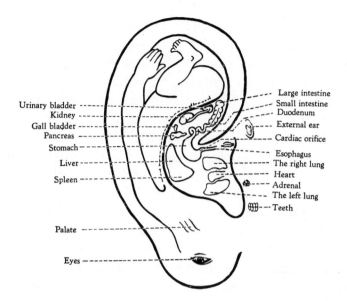

Corresponding Regional Anatomy of the Auricular Points and Fetus

illnesses that can be treated by stimulating points on the feet. The hands are also an energetic microcosm of the body. Bronchitis and malaria are two of the illnesses that can be treated through stimulating points on the hands. The practice of palm reading is said to have ancient roots in health care. Although I am not sure that "reading" a palm is a microcosmic view of a person's destiny, I *do* know that by simply observing the shape of your hands and fingers, as well as the lines on your palm, an energetic therapist can tell you a lot about the current state of your health—and possibly its future state as well.

I think the slow acceptance of acupuncture in the

West is mainly due to the fact that most Westerners strongly associate needles with pain, instead of with relief from it. In the past few decades, promotional photographs of patients being treated with hundreds of needles have left indelible, frightening images in many Westerner's minds. These attempts at promoting acupuncture in the West have actually hurt the cause, and prevented many people who would greatly benefit from treatment from seeking help. I tend to hear the same fears about acupuncture again and again. Let me assure you: Acupuncture is a very safe, very effective, natural way of both preventing and curing many illnesses. It is not painful. Usually fewer than ten needles are used in one treatment, and all needles are disposable—the same needle is *never* used again on another patient. Treatments generally last from twenty to forty minutes, and are very relaxing. Afterward the patient usually experiences a feeling of lightness and general well-being. While results are often seen immediately, complete healing is usually the result of a series of treatments given over a period of weeks, months, or sometimes even years.

There are some Westerners who discount the success of acupuncture as being a kind of "placebo" effect; that is, results are realized only because the patient *believes* it will cure them. Although the mind is an extremely powerful part of the healing process, as we will see in the next chapter, the amazing healing powers of acupuncture are very real. It works whether or not the person fully believes in the technique, and it forms a critical type of health care millions of people rely upon all over the world, especially in the East and in Europe.

As further proof of its effectiveness, look at the successful use of acupuncture in veterinary medicine. Complex energy networks have been plotted in many animals, including dogs, cats, and horses. Animals, lacking our level of consciousness, do not have any *expectations* of relief from acupuncture. Yet acupuncture has an 80 percent success rate in treating animals. A dog that could not walk on a painful leg walks perfectly normally after treatment, and there is no doubt that the animal's quality of life has most definitely improved.

Q.M. therapy is another energetic healing technique offered at the Q.M. Institute. Instead of focusing on just the twelve primary channels and two governing vessels, Q.M. therapy engages all of the patient's energy system at once. It is a technique in which the energetic therapist uses his or her own energy to rebalance the energy in the patient's system. Becoming a Q.M. therapist takes many years of dedicated study, because the therapist must be very aware not only of how every channel works, but also of how they work together in their many combinations. In order to accomplish this, he or she must be familiar with *every* channel in the body, the entire energy system.

When treating a patient, a Q.M. therapist must first reach a very high level of mental concentration. Next comes "scanning," which is passing a hand over the patient's body to sense the exact location of the energy blockage or imbalance. Now the therapist must determine the exact *type* of energy that is blocked—not just which of the five phases, but also the exact level of energy within that phase. Once this is accomplished, the therapist must call up the exact type of healing energy, the appropriate creative or controlling energy, in himself. Using intense mental concentration alone, this energy is passed through to the patient's body. Many times this is accomplished *without* physically touching the patient at all. In fact, in some cases a highly trained Q.M. therapist can successfully manipulate a patient's energy from across the room!

As you are just beginning to feel and understand your own energy, it may seem unbelievable to you that someone could actually feel five distinct levels of it. Actually, highly qualified energetic therapists who practice this technique can feel many more than that. They are true energy experts. There is absolutely no guesswork involved. They have mastered their own energy to the point where they can feel and manipulate not only the energy within themselves, but also the energy within others. When it comes to energy, they can be viewed as extraordinarily sensitive and perceptive people. As you progress in your quest to control your own energy, you, too, will able to feel its different qualities.

Although I have often used the Q.M. technique in my own practice, I usually only employ it as a last resort because of the high level of concentration I must reach in order to perform it. While I can treat a few people in an hour using acupuncture needles, with Q.M. therapy I can only treat one person at a time. And as I am using my own energy, instead of needles, to rebalance the patient's energy, I become physically exhausted, completely drained, by the end of the day. But in some cases there is no other alternative. I once treated a woman suffering from a terrible disease called scleroderma, where the skin becomes very hard and any kind of touch is painful. It was impossible to even penetrate her skin with hair-thin acupuncture needles. But using Q.M. therapy, I was able to engage and rebalance her energy system without touching her, and her condition quickly improved.

Although Q.M. therapy is often compared to hands-on psychic healing, it is actually a much more refined and effective practice. Psychic healing has proven to be effective at times, but it still has not been scientifically studied enough to be thoroughly understood. Q.M. therapy is a scientific, proven method that has been developed over thousands of years. Its methods are refined; it is a scientific approach to healing that requires extensive training and study.

No matter what technique is used, balancing all the inner energy of the human body requires almost constant effort. It can be compared to the struggle we used to face in getting a good picture on our televisions: We constantly play with the antenna and adjust the vertical hold, the horizontal hold, and all the other knobs until we get our perfect picture, or a balanced energy system. Soon new interference sets in and the image begins to gets "snowy"; our energy system becomes unbalanced, and we start all over again.

The human body is a very complex instrument that is continually struggling to "stay in tune," or balance its many different inner energies. Think of an energetic therapist as an accomplished conductor who is able to "tune" a 120-piece symphony orchestra. The tuning process begins with the tuning of each individual instrument, then of each section of instruments, then of the entire orchestra together. As each instrument or section is tuned, the vibrations throw the rest of the section—and then the rest of the orchestra—*out* of tune. After a lot of fine adjustments you finally get a sound you can live with. Think how long it takes just to tune a six-string guitar. Now imagine the task of tuning an entire symphony orchestra! This is what the energetic therapist faces—and accomplishes. He or she is constantly trying to find the most effective energetic treatment for each patient.

Keeping our bodies "in tune" is something we all struggle to do. Every second of our lives we strive to balance the air energy we breathe with the energies we obtain from eating, drinking, and exercising. There is no single way to keep your energy system in balance. Chapters 5 and 6 will show you how to balance all of your inner energies by following a basic energetic health program that includes general guidelines for a balanced lifestyle.

You now have a basic understanding of how energy works in your body—but this is still only half the picture. The next step is to understand the energy potential contained in your mind, the second part of the critical *yin* and *yang* relationship that comprises your entire being. Once you understand how your physical being interacts with your emotional and spiritual being, you will fully understand your own extraordinary power—a power that can heal both yourself and others—and you will understand how to use that power to improve every facet of your life.

Chapter Four

ENERGETICS: BODY, MIND, AND SPIRIT

OUR BODY, mind, and spirit represent three basic levels of energy that comprise our total existence, and our energy constantly moves through all three of these levels. Each level must be in balanced harmony with the other two in order for both physical and mental health to be realized. An energy imbalance within any level will upset the balance of the other two. Of the three levels, our body's energy is the easiest to study, simply because specific energy pathways have been "mapped out." We have been able to trace the patterns or channels of this energy and therefore understand how to control it. Even though we cannot see the actual energy, most people experience it in the same way. So an acupuncture needle placed at the same point will affect almost every patient who responds to treatment in exactly the same way.

But the energy that comprises the next level of our

existence is much more difficult to study. The nature of our mind's energy is more elusive; it cannot be "drawn," cannot be captured in a simple illustration. So it is more difficult for everyone to agree exactly how this level of energy works. Yet, just as the pattern of energy channels that runs through our bodies was painstakingly located through trial and error over centuries of research and study, so, too, has a second overall pattern been located. This second pattern shows that the mind's energy and the body's energy system interact in very specific ways. The relationship between mind and body energy forms many distinct patterns that recur in patient after patient. As we begin our discussion of the mind's energy, it is important to understand that this includes both the energy of our conscious awareness and that of our subconscious self. As you will see in this chapter, both the thoughts and emotions we are aware of *and* those we are not aware of powerfully affect the status of our health.

In many ways, the mind is the essence of our being. It rules the body's energy system and is the most powerful healing tool we have. The mind is the center of willpower, and willpower directs the life energy that flows through our bodies. Just as thought can be used to contract or relax any individual muscle at will (including "involuntary" muscles), thought can also be developed to direct our energy to heal any part of the body. As I discussed in the previous chapter, our energy is not just energy, but energy *plus* information. By concentrating on a particular portion of the body, we can send energy there—energy that literally delivers a message. For example, mental concentration can be developed to stop nervous heart palpitations, control pain, or destroy a cancerous tumor. And just as the brain alerts us to a disruption of energy flow in the body, it can also work to rebalance the energy, whether by manufacturing and releasing chemicals, blocking neural impulses that carry a "pain" message to the brain, or increasing the number of cancer-fighting white blood cells. Mental energy can control both the direction of energy flowing in our energy channels and the *exact form* (phase) the flow of energy will take.

The power of the mind is finally being accepted, recognized, and studied in Western science. In *The Body Electric*, Dr. Becker described his findings, which showed that hypnotized patients can actually produce voltage changes in specific parts of the body upon command. Western science is currently using these results as a possible explanation for the placebo effect discussed in the last chapter, and for hypnosis cures.

The mind's energy, our willpower, can be developed to control our body's energy system to an extraordinary degree. You can learn to direct energy through any specific energy channel simply by *thinking* about it, by sending energy there with your mind. This may sound more advanced to you than it actually is. The previously discussed examples of "zoning" illustrated an advanced state of consciousness, of energy control. Turning this power on and off takes years of practice and training to achieve. But you don't have to wait that long. You can start experiencing the power of your mind right now.

At the beginning of chapter 2, I asked you to touch

the center of your palms to locate the two energy centers there. Rubbing your hands together for a few minutes activated these centers and warmed your entire body. Now you are going to do the same thing—but this time using only your mind.

Find a quiet place and sit with your back straight and both feet on the floor. As you begin to relax, turn your palms to face upward on your lap. Now shut your eyes and imagine a red circle at the center of each palm. Let all the tension flow out of your body as you concentrate your mind's energy on these two red spots. After a minute or so of reaching a relaxed state of concentration, imagine the red areas becoming brighter and more intense. After a few more minutes, you will feel a gentle pulsing sensation in each palm as your mind activates both energy centers. Soon this gentle pulsation will give rise to a feeling of warmth that will begin to spread all over your body.

This exercise may require a few tries, but with continued practice you will eventually be able to warm your body just as effectively as when you physically rub your hands together.

Although the mind's energy can be developed to direct and control the body's energy, don't forget that mind and body coexist in a *yin/yang* relationship—so an energy imbalance in one creates an energy imbalance in the other. While the mind can be used to prevent illness and promote healing, an emotional imbalance within the mind can also *create* illness. Most people today agree that chronic anxiety can create ulcers—but ulcers can also create chronic anxiety. Emotions are simply expressions of your mind's energy. And just as your mind and emotions act directly upon your body's energy system, so does your body's energy system directly affect your mind and emotional balance. For example, constantly feeling angry over a period of time can upset the balance of energy in your liver channel. And, similarly, a chronic energy imbalance in the liver channel, caused by an improper diet, for example, can make you feel irritable and angry. Illness can begin in either the mind or the body. And true healing cannot take place until both are balanced.

Emotions are, of course, a natural part of life. They are the blend of mind and senses. An emotion will only negatively affect the energy balance that governs your health when it is either excessive or deficient over a long period of time, or when it arises very suddenly with a great deal of force. Just as a sudden movement can sprain an ankle, or excessive use of one part of the body can create a physical imbalance, the same holds true for our emotions. Again, balance is always the key to health.

Seven principle emotions are considered to have the most important impact on your body's energy: anger, joy, sadness, grief, worry, fear, and fright. Each of these seven basic emotions directly impacts the twelve primary energy channels (although the heart and liver energy channels are considered the most vulnerable to emotional disturbance). Each emotion is a primary factor in the disease process—that is, in the process of producing an energy imbalance (See table 4). But again, don't take the seven basic emotions too literally. There are many different levels to each, and the same emotion doesn't always affect every person exactly the same way. Each is just another general sign the energetic therapist can use to determine the pattern of disharmony.

As you read through the following discussion of the seven principle emotions, it may be helpful to refer back to the energy channel illustrations in the last chapter.

TABLE 4

PHASE:	Wood	Fire	Earth	Metal	Water
SEASON:	Spring	Summer	Late summer	Autumn	Winter
YIN CHANNEL:	Liver	Heart	Spleen	Lungs	Kidney
YANG CHANNEL:	Gall bladder	Small intestine, Triple burner, Pericardium	Stomach	Large intestine	Bladder
EMOTION:	Anger	Joy	Worry	Sadness, Grief	Fear, Fright
EXCESS EMOTION:	Rising energy	Slow, scattered energy	"Stuck" energy	Weak energy	Chaotic energy
DISHARMONY SEEN IN:	Eyes, Nails	Tongue, Facial complexion	Mouth, Lips	Nose, Skin	Ears, Hair

Anger.

Associated with the "wood" phase of energy, anger is often described as an "explosive" emotion. It is similar to the type of energy seen in the spring season. In spring, flowers bloom to create an "explosion" of color.

Thunderstorms often include explosive bursts of rain. The energy of anger is the energy of sudden, powerful activity.

I think anger is one of the most problematic emotions in Western society because of the cultural pressure to deny its very existence. For Westerners, it is often considered rude to display anger or discuss it in any way. And anger can take many forms: resentment, depression (anger turned against oneself), prolonged frustration, or bitterness. Any of these can affect the energy that flows through the liver and gall bladder channels.

Excess anger causes energy to rise like heat in the body, often resulting in an angry person's bright red face. Chronic poor vision or a variety of eye problems and brittle nails are two of the most common signs of a liver or gall bladder channel imbalance caused by or associated with excess anger.

Because the liver channel is responsible for harmonizing all the emotions and overseeing the smooth flow of energy throughout the body, anger can have a devastating effect on the body's overall energy system, increasing the likelihood of developing a wide variety of diseases, including cancer. Anger also affects the digestive process because it increases the amount of energy in the liver channel. When this happens, energy can "spill over" into the spleen and stomach channels. Energy that moves in the wrong direction in the liver channel can be the result of or source of excessive anger. Stagnated energy in this channel may be associated with emotional frustration or with inappropriate and extreme mood changes.

The gall bladder channel is said to rule our decision-making abilities. Excess anger may lead to an energy imbalance in this channel, which could cause one to make poor or rash decisions. When we say someone "has a lot of gall" we are actually referring to excess energy in this channel. We are usually describing disruptive or "nervy" behavior, and it is this energy that is motivating the person's angry actions. On the other hand, too little energy in this channel can result in indecision and timidity, and may also signify gall bladder disharmony.

Anger is a powerful emotion that upsets the energy balance in a variety of ways. In addition to the illnesses previously mentioned, excess anger, over time, can cause dizziness, high blood pressure, muscle spasms, ulcers, colitis, and irritable bowel syndrome. Anger can also literally create "a bitter taste in one's mouth."

Joy.

Joy is associated with fire energy, with the warmth and activity typical of summer. A joyful person is said to be a "warm" person, and is often busy doing things for others. Fire energy is also expansive energy. Feelings of joy actually expand, like warmth spreading throughout the body. In fact, joy is often said to be "contagious"— that is, able to spread from person to person.

Joy is primarily associated with the energy that runs through the heart channel, which is said to house the spirit. We will be discussing our spiritual energy later in the chapter; for now, you simply need to know that this higher level of energy most directly affects this channel. When we say someone has "a big heart," we are referring to the high level of energy that runs through this channel and nourishes the person's vitality, their spirit. Saying that someone has "a heavy heart" refers to depleted energy in this channel and describes someone whose spirit is weak.

It may be difficult for you to believe that being *too* happy could ever be a problem, but it can. We cry not only when we are overly sad, but when we are overly happy as well, and constant excess joy can negatively affect our health. Too much continual excitement can drain this energy and cause slow, scattered energy to flow throughout the small intestine, triple burner, and pericardium channels as well. Because most of these channels run up to and around the head area, signs of an energy imbalance caused by excess joy are often seen in the tongue and facial complexion. Too much joy can unbalance your energy and lead to a variety of problems, including muddled thinking, inappropriate laughing or crying, heart palpitations, insomnia, stiff neck, abdominal pain, and a feeling of tightness in the chest.

Worry.

People who worry too much are people who spend too much time thinking and too little time doing. They are standing still emotionally, partially paralyzed. This is why worry is associated with the earth phase of energy. It is the energy of neutrality and balance, creating the illusion of standing still (although this is, of course, only an illusion; energy may slow down enough to appear to stop moving, but it never actually does). "Earth" energy is the energy of maturity, of adulthood, and adults usually worry much more than children. It is the energy of late summer, when crops are harvested, when nature's growth cycle has peaked.

Worrying too much drains the energy that runs through the spleen and stomach channels. Students, overwrought executives, and others experiencing excessive worry often suffer from a loss of appetite and insomnia. Worrying too much causes the body's energy to stagnate in both of these channels. Unbalanced energy in the spleen channel reduces its ability to transform food into energy, resulting in poor digestion or stomach distention. Because the energy in the spleen channel also regulates the body's blood supply, "stuck" energy caused by worry in this channel can result in anemia, menstrual problems, chronic hepatitis, and fatigue. Stagnated energy in the stomach channel may disrupt the body's ability to take in food, and can result in nausea and vomiting in addition to loss of appetite.

Sadness and Grief.

The emotions of sadness and grief (excessive sadness) are manifestations of metal energy. This is the energy of autumn: The leaves that grew on the trees dry up and fall to the ground as earth energy gives rise to metal energy. The emotions associated with this type of energy, be it autumn or "old age," are often feelings associated with loss.

When it comes to our own beings, excess sadness and grief weaken the energy that runs through the lung and large intestine channels. These emotions may also affect the energy that runs through the heart channel, which in turn will weaken the spirit. Because the lung channel oversees the body's intake of air as well as the entire energy system, weak energy in this channel caused by sadness can result in coughing, asthma, allergies, skin problems, bronchitis, and fatigue. Other physical symptoms may include extreme lethargy and shortness of breath. Weak energy in the large intestine channel often results in a distended abdomen, constipation, and diarrhea. In some cases, illnesses related to the blood may also appear. Children of divorce, for example, often experience overwhelming sadness and grief over the loss of their family's unity, and are frequently afflicted with asthma and other illnesses associated with these powerful emotions.

Fear and Fright.

Fear and fright (excessive fear) are the emotions associated with water energy, the energy that both concludes and begins the life cycle. Water energy is often associated with change, and fear and fright often accompany two of the greatest changes we all experience—birth and death. Water energy is fluid, moving energy, and is often associated with chaos. In fact, fear of change and fear of chaos are two fears most of us share.

In the body, fear and fright are associated with chaotic energy that mainly upsets the energy balance within the kidney and bladder channels. Fear in young children often results in weak kidney energy that leads to bedwetting. Energy imbalances caused by fear are often reflected in a patient's hair, and fright can even create "hair-raising" sensations. But these extremely powerful emotions can also create such chaotic energetic activity that a wide range of physical ailments can result, including a variety of ear problems. Because the kidney

channel stores the body's reproductive energy, repressed fear of being pregnant and the responsibility
of parenthood can often prevent a seemingly enthusi-
astic couple from conceiving a child. Once the fear is
uncovered and worked out, pregnancy often quickly
follows.

Just as the seven primary emotions relate to the five
phases, they also exist in similar creating and controlling relationships (see figure 19).

Whether we are aware of them or not, we all have
these seven basic emotions. It may be difficult to understand the complex relationships that exist among them,
and discussing them in detail is beyond the scope of this
book. The important thing to understand is that it is
normal to experience all of these emotions, and that as
long as they co-exist in balanced harmony, they will not
cause any health problems. But when there is too much
or too little of one emotion, our entire emotional and
physical state of being can be thrown off balance.

It may be difficult to understand how the emotions
create one another—for example, how anger "feeds" joy.
But properly getting in touch with your anger and releasing it does, indeed, lead to happiness. And while the
proper level of joy in our lives keeps anger and worry in
balance, the right amount of worry, so to speak, also
balances out joy and sadness. The same holds true for
the controlling relationships. Using these charts as a
general guideline for emotional balance, understand
that the proper amount of anger will keep worry or
concern in balance. The right amount of worry or concern will control the feeling of fear, and so on. It is

FIGURE 19

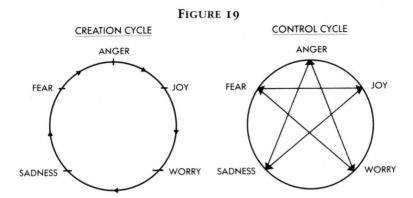

CREATION CYCLE

ANGER

FEER   JOY

SADNESS   WORRY

CONTROL CYCLE

ANGER

FEAR   JOY

SADNESS   WORRY

important not to repress emotions. This is a tremendous waste of energy, and will deplete your entire energy system. Emotions must continually be properly released in order to maintain a healthy emotional balance.

The mind constantly strives to maintain our emotional balance. Thought *is* energy, and also *directs* our total energy, including our physical energy and our emotional energy. Emotions are often described as being "powerful." In order to be and stay healthy, we must learn to control this power. The first step in accomplishing this is to realize and accept the fact that you *choose* your emotions. Nothing "makes" you feel anything. You choose to react to situations and people with particular emotions. For example, some people choose to feel fear when flying in an airplane while others choose to feel joy. The exact same activity is experienced in opposite ways. The same holds true when reacting to people. No one can "make" you feel happy or sad. While it is true that miserable people can be "draining" to be around—which may indeed cause you to feel miserable as well—by allowing yourself to be miserable you are still choosing to feel miserable, as well as choosing to spend time with that person.

Thought energy actually travels in resonating waves. It is energy that flows from the mind into the universe. Just as your physical energy travels from your hands to warm the glass you are holding, thought energy also affects everything around you, and vice versa. Pressing a key on a piano produces a sound by causing one of the piano's strings to vibrate, thus propagating energy through the air in the form of "sound" vibrations. When that same note is played higher on the scale, the sound waves occur at a higher frequency and a crystal vase on the piano could begin to vibrate. Played at an even higher pitch, that same note could actually cause that vase to shatter. The vibrational energy of each sound caused a different type of sympathetic vibrational response in the vase.

The same thing happens with the thoughts that resonate from your mind into your body. Your thoughts also send out vibrational energy that causes sympathetic responses in your body. Just as a high note may shatter a crystal vase, a strong negative emotion such as grief, experienced consciously or not, may "strike a similar chord" in your physical being, resulting in a severe asthmatic attack. Your mental energy affects the minds and objects around you, as well, to varying degrees depending on its strength. Therefore, it is important to realize that negative thoughts send destructive energy not only throughout your body, but throughout the universe as well, affecting everything around you.

Although understanding the patterns of harmony and

disharmony that govern your body and mind energies is essential to finding your own life balance, you cannot understand your total energetic being without an awareness of your third and highest level of energy, your spiritual energy. This level of energy is even more elusive, more difficult to comprehend than the mind's energy. When we attempt to determine the nature of someone's spirit, we are trying to determine the level of that person's overall vitality, the amount of enthusiasm one has for one's own life—or, simply put, one's desire to live.

Spiritual energy may be described as the energy associated with "higher consciousness," or the "enlightenment" that is found at the *mahat* level of energy in the ancient Indian tradition. Although less is known about this level of energy than about the other two, patterns of disharmony between spirit, body, and mind have been found as well. As previously discussed, the strength or weakness of our spiritual energy directly impacts the heart channel in our body's energy system—the channel which "rules the head and houses the spirit," and is associated with the emotion of joy. Strong, steady spiritual energy will keep this energy channel in balance and maintain proper circulation of blood throughout the body. But excess or weak spiritual energy can create problems.

Excess, uncontrolled spiritual energy can lead to excess joy, which can then slow down and dissipate energy throughout much of the body, leaving behind a wake of symptoms, including insomnia and muddled thinking. On the other hand, insufficient spiritual energy depletes the energy in the heart channel. The resulting lack of joy gives rise to excess sadness and grief. Like falling dominoes, these emotions affect other channels which in turn give rise to other excess emotions. Soon the body's entire energy system may be devastated. This may be referred to as "dying from a broken heart."

The eyes have been called the "windows to the soul," and, indeed, just by looking someone in the eye you can learn a lot about how they feel about his or her own life. This important sign of people's overall well-being is often described as "the light" in their eyes. How bright that light is shows how strong or weak their spiritual energy is. "Shining" or "sparkling" eyes, or "a twinkle" in the eye, are signs of a healthy spirit. On the other hand, a "dark look" or a "dullness" in someone's eyes is a sign of depleted spiritual energy. If you refer back to the illustration in chapter 2, showing the heart channel, you will see something interesting. The channel flows upward and stops directly in the center of each eye. Just as your mind's energy can be concentrated to engage and control your body's energy, so can you "raise" your consciousness through mental concentration to engage and control the spiritual level of your energy. This is achieved through meditation.

In its effort to study the mind and "higher consciousness," modern science has begun to study how the brain itself works. The results of this study continue to validate the ancient views on energy that underlie all energetic medicine. So far, research has found that our brains give off faint electrical impulses which can be measured. Different types of these brain waves were found to move at different rates. When we sleep, our brain activity slows down as consciousness gives way to allow the body to heal and repair itself. There is a powerful energy release as natural healing processes automatically become active throughout the body. These slower vibrations that occur during sleep are called delta waves. When electrical activity slightly increases to the theta wave level, we are in a lighter stage of sleep, deeply relaxed, drowsy, or in a state of creativity. Alpha waves are even faster and occur during lighter relaxed states. When we are in an alert, conscious state, different brain waves operate together in various combinations at even faster rates. But research has proven that during meditation the brain operates in a completely different way. As consciousness is used to calm the mind and relax the body, a light trance state is reached—yet brain wave activity *increases*. And the brain waves themselves start to move in a more orderly, synchronized fashion.

In addition to the increased orderliness of the brain's electrical activity, two other primary changes take place during meditation: The body's metabolic rate slows way down, and the nervous system automatically balances itself. Much of the scientific knowledge we have about what happens to the body during meditation is the result of a groundbreaking study by physiologist Robert Keith Wallace. In 1970, he published the results of the first major study of the effects of meditation on the body during the first twenty minutes of practice.* His findings startled the scientific community.

* Harold H. Blumfield, M.D., and Robert B. Korg, *Happiness—TM Program: Psychiatry and Enlightenment* (New York: Simon and Schuster: 1976).

Dr. Wallace studied thirty-six men and women of different ages who had been practicing transcendental meditation (TM) for various lengths of time. TM is a meditative program with ancient roots in the Indian tradition. Each subject was monitored for basic bodily functions. Wallace found that dramatic changes occurred within each of the thirty-six people. The most startling was that each person reached a unique state of consciousness that provided *more* rest than the deepest point of sleep.

The principal way to measure a person's level of activity or rest is by how much oxygen, or air energy, he or she is consuming over a period of time. Running requires a higher oxygen intake than sitting, sitting requires more oxygen than sleeping, and so on. After five or six hours of being asleep your oxygen intake drops to a level 8 to 10 percent lower than when you're awake. But Wallace found that after just a few minutes of meditation, oxygen intake drops 16 to 18 percent—almost twice the drop acquired through deep sleep. The dramatic drop in oxygen intake during consciousness showed that meditation allows the body to operate on a much more efficient level. While retaining consciousness, meditation puts the mind into a unique, deeply relaxed state.

In late 1972, neurophysiologist J. P. Banquet found that TM also *unified* brain wave activity.* He discovered that TM produced a unique state of consciousness that combines theta waves, those waves associated with

* Harold H. Blumfield, M.D., and Robert B. Korg, *Happiness—TM Program: Psychiatry and Enlightenment* (New York: Simon and Schuster: 1976).

deep relaxation, with alpha waves, the brain wave activity of active consciousness. Banquet found that after a few minutes of TM, the brain's alpha waves began to move in a synchronized fashion from the back of the brain to the front and between the left and right hemispheres. And the electrical activity not only balanced itself, but also remained in this state for varying lengths of time *after* the meditation was over. Since the 1970s, dozens of other studies have shown that regular meditation, whether TM or any of a number of other techniques, increased general concentration, improved self-esteem, and decreased depression and anxiety. Meditators have been found to decrease their use of alcohol, cigarettes, and tranquilizers, and to stop overeating.

As I mentioned earlier, new sciences like psychoneuroimmunology, the study of the mind's ability to control the body's immune system, are showing that meditation can be used not only to prevent illness, but also to treat even terminal illnesses like cancer. One of Western medicine's most widely accepted explanations for cancer, the "surveillance theory," states that cancer cells are developing within us all the time, but are destroyed by white blood cells before they can develop into dangerous tumors. Cancer appears when the immune system becomes suppressed and can no longer deal with this routine threat. Furthermore, recent research has revealed that there is actually an anatomical link between the brain and the immune system. Our immune system consists of more than a dozen different types of white blood cells, concentrated in the spleen, thymus gland, and lymph nodes, which patrol the entire body through the blood and lymphatic systems. Researchers have discovered nerves that connect the thymus and spleen directly to the hypothalamus, a tiny part of the brain that regulates most of the body's unconscious maintenance processes such as heartbeat, breathing, blood pressure, and temperature.

Western science has also found "visual" evidence of the link between mind energy and body energy. Two of the most renowned innovators in this field are oncologist O. Carl Simonton and psychologist Stephanie Matthews-Simonton. The Simontons conducted a study in which they had cancer patients meditate three times a day for fifteen minutes. Before each meditation the patients were shown pictures of their cancers, whether they be tumors or lesions, being destroyed— that is, pictures of white blood cells fighting cancer cells. During their meditation the cancer patients were asked to first visualize their particular lesion or tumor. Then they pictured the tumor cells in their bodies as dead or dying, with the white blood cells swarming over the tumors, destroying the cancer cells and carrying them off. At the end of the meditation, the patients were asked to visualize themselves free of disease and in perfect health. In their first study of 159 terminal cancer cases (all expected to die within one year), 41 percent of the patients showed remarkable improvement: in 22 percent of those studied the cancer began to recede, and in 19 percent it *completely disappeared.* The remaining 59 percent of the patients, who did eventually die from the disease, lived an average of twice as long as they were expected to.

Studies have also shown that the body cannot be

outsmarted. Imagery does not work if the patient is in denial. Pretending that disease doesn't exist does not get rid of the disease. The patient must first visualize the disease and then truly believe it to be destroyed in order for healing to take place. The body only knows what the mind tells it.

Different meditative techniques work for different people. Some do well with structured programs like TM, while others design their own. But no matter what works best for you, meditation should become a part of your daily life. You can use it to soothe your mind and heal both body and spirit. By simply focusing your mind's energy, you not only harmonize all three levels of your energetic existence, but also unify yourself and the universe by balancing your inner energy with that of the world around you. Meditation should be practiced for at least fifteen minutes each day, alone, in a quiet place. Begin each session by closing your eyes, relaxing your body, and taking deep breaths. Think of the air you breathe in as the outer energy that becomes your inner energy, revitalizes it, and then goes back out. Focus on the rhythm of your breathing as you repeat a simple positive affirmation. Meditation is a simple way to engage all three levels of your energy, and a powerful tool at your constant disposal to strengthen your spiritual energy and maintain your overall vitality.

Observing your spirit and emotions is one of the first things an energetic therapist will do when examining you. Western physicians, however, are not trained to do so. Since the spirit cannot be seen directly nor thoughts measured (unless, of course, you know what to look for) Western medicine tends to ignore half of your being.

Western medicine *does* often recognize what is called psychosomatic illness—that is, illness triggered by an emotional problem. Yet because we cannot "see" our emotions, these very real illnesses are still thought to be somewhat unreal—even when the physical manifestations are clearly visible. Energetic medicine, because it emphasizes the balance of the "whole" person, can frequently discover and treat an illness before it can be detected by even the most sophisticated Western diagnostic techniques. It is clear that human beings consist of more than the eye can see, and energetic medicine has always recognized the complex relationships that exist between mind, body, and spirit. It takes into account the totality of our human reality. Our spirit, mind, and emotions are considered to be as real as our physical bodies, and are recognized to interact in very specific ways.

As previously discussed, specific emotions actually affect specific energy channels. Therefore, by rebalancing the energy within these affected channels, the emotions themselves are rebalanced—*and* vice versa. Chronic anger as a reaction to stress can create a chronic energy imbalance in the liver channel. In order to correct it, the energetic therapist can rebalance the body's energy, and the patient will actually stop feeling angry—at least until a stressful situation is experienced again. That's why complete healing will only occur when both body and mind are treated. Negative thoughts and emotions are almost always the root of any illness. Although the body's energy can be rebalanced constantly with an energetic treatment, until a patient prone to anger finds a healthier way to cope with stress, the imbalance will continue to occur.

When treating an illness, an energetic therapist first has to determine exactly *what* is triggering the energy imbalance. Is the patient's illness primarily the result of unbalanced emotional energy, or of an energy imbalance in the body? Is the patient's diet the cause of the illness? Then why is the patient choosing to eat foods that are literally making him or her sick? The solution to the mystery of each patient's illness is always a combination of many factors. Each part of the patient's life must be taken into account in order to rebalance the person's complete energy system. Each illness is a puzzle with many pieces. The energetic therapist must first collect all these pieces and then put them together. Only then will he or she be able to find the pattern of disharmony and be able to *alter* that pattern. This can be a complicated, difficult task. Solving the mystery of each patient's illness is like taking a trip with him— exploring his life to find out what is out of balance. As you will see in the following cases from my private practice, it is also a fascinating process.

Case Study # I

One very humid August morning, Catherine, a woman in her late twenties, a successful television producer, walked into my office and sat down across from me. Observing the way she walked, I noticed slightly stooped shoulders and a slow hesitation about where she should sit. Although Catherine was smiling, I noticed her underlying demeanor to be somewhat sad, and there was a nervousness about her—all signs of a weak spirit. Since the age of thirteen she had experienced somewhat severe edema—periodic swelling in her ankles and feet and occasional water retention throughout her entire body. The problem had now become chronic and worsened in the humid weather we were having that day. She had seen a variety of Western doctors, who all told her there was nothing to be done about her condition. And so she came to me.

As we talked about her symptoms, Catherine told me the swelling became worse in severe humidity and practically disappeared in the winter. As I listened to her describe her symptoms I again noticed that her manner was very subdued. As we talked, she said she led an active life and thought things were going very well in general. Checking her pulses, I noticed a tight, floating pulse that pointed to an energy imbalance in the lung channel, a sinking pulse associated with the spleen channel, and a frail pulse in the kidney channel. Her tongue was slightly swollen, surrounded by ridges, and had a thin white coating. The color of the tongue itself was a bit pale. Other signs were a sallow complexion, swollen eyelids, and cold hands and feet.

Putting these signs and symptoms together, the energy imbalances in her lung, spleen, and kidney channels clearly formed a pattern of disharmony of excess water energy throughout her system, what Western medicine would simply call edema. After a forty-minute acupuncture treatment that rebalanced the energy in these channels by increasing her fire energy, the swelling practically disappeared right before our eyes—even on this humid day. But a few days later the condition returned, and she came back for her second treatment.

This time we discussed the possible emotions that

may have been part of the mystery of her illness. Catherine said she liked her job very much even though it
was extremely stressful. But she felt she could handle it
well because she grew up in a violent household and was
"used to stress." I told her that her physical condition
pointed to a lot of repressed anger. She said she didn't
feel angry, but did suffer from periodic bouts of depression. After we discussed it further, she agreed to go for
counseling in addition to coming for more acupuncture
treatments. Within six months her condition improved
tremendously. She was finally getting in touch with all
the anger she had always held back, the anger she didn't
even know she had. In addition to her predisposition to
edema, her emotional nature (a tendency to hold in all
her emotions) sent a message to each and every cell of
her body to hold in water. On top of that she aggravated
her condition by eating a lot of salty junk food and fried
foods, and by not exercising. As Catherine's counselor
helped her gradually release her anger and find a better
way to react to stress, she continued to come to me for
treatment. Soon her edema started to disappear for
good. Catherine also changed her diet and started an
exercise program, and her edema was almost completely gone within a year.

Case Study # II

A patient's symptoms don't always lead right to the pattern of disharmony. David, a busy executive in his early
thirties, came to see me complaining of general fatigue.
His regular doctor had not been able to find anything
physically wrong with him. He said that nothing in his

life had changed recently, so he could not understand his sudden state of exhaustion. His spirit seemed strong but I noticed that he spoke very quickly, sometimes getting red in the face.

Taking David's pulses, I found a tight pulse in his lung channel and a wiry pulse that is associated with the liver channel. These two imbalances in the channels that oversee the entire system explained his fatigue. His tongue looked dry, with a thin white coating (indicating a build up of toxic wastes in the stomach). All of these signs, together with his red eyes, slightly red face, and hurried, irritable nature, pointed to a pattern of disharmony that often produces recurrent headaches. I asked him if he had been getting headaches lately, and he seemed surprised that he had somehow forgotten to mention that he had. He then started coughing, and told me he had suffered from asthma since he was a child, and sometimes had to take medication.

Although David assured me his life was fine, that he was successful and happy in his new marriage, something was clearly going wrong—something that was depleting the energy in his entire system. I asked him about the family he grew up in. He said his parents divorced when he was a child and his mother has always been emotionally dependent on him. He and his new wife had just bought a house, but had to borrow the down payment because he now supported his mother financially as well.

From his physical signs I could tell that David was actually very angry inside, but didn't know it. After an acupuncture treatment that increased and rebalanced his body's energy he felt much better, but I knew the problem would return until he worked out his relationship with his mother. During his next scheduled treatment I asked him how his mother was doing. He told me she was driving him crazy, constantly creating situations which he felt forced him to be at her house all the time for one reason or another. The situation was putting pressure on both his home life and career. Finally he said, "She's suffocating me." Since he had ignored his feelings, his body had to deliver the message. The suffocation he felt as a child manifested itself literally as asthma. That energy-draining relationship had not been corrected and was now draining his entire system. As David became more aware of the problem over the next six months, he gradually set limits on how much time he spent with his mother. After some initial anger she lessened her dependence on him, joined some organizations, and made some friends. David's chronic fatigue soon disappeared, and both his and his mother's overall lives improved.

Case Study #III

Acute pain in the back of the right and left shoulders brought a third patient to see me. Terry was a woman in her early forties, a busy executive in a publishing company. She said she had simply woken up two days before with the condition. She was now in so much pain she could hardly move either shoulder. She said she had not strained her back, and had no idea why this had happened.

A frail pulse told me there were energy imbalances in the lung and large intestine channels. Terry's tongue was pale, another sign of a problem in the large intestine. When I examined her I quickly felt that both shoulders were completely frozen; the muscles were so tense that they were hard as rocks. I found an acupuncture point on the large intestine channel on her right shoulder. It was right in the middle of a very stiff muscle. As I applied gentle pressure to this point and began to rotate her shoulder Terry suddenly burst into tears. She was so overwhelmed that she could not stop sobbing. When I asked her what was wrong she said she hadn't realized until just now that this day was the first anniversary of her brother's death. The overwhelming grief that she had been keeping inside created a severe energy blockage in the large intestine channel. By simply rubbing an energy point on the channel and releasing this blocked energy, I was able to help her release her grief. Terry was still in mourning for her brother's death and just had to let herself cry. She took some time off from work to confront her grief and within two days the pain in both shoulders completely disappeared.

Case Study #IV

Sometimes treating a patient begins with treating a patient's spouse. Once, one of my associates, one of the most accomplished Q.M. therapists I knew, came in to see me. I could see how upset he was before he even said a word. I knew his wife had been suffering from diabetes for years and that he had been treating her quite successfully with Q.M. therapy. But now he told me that in the past few weeks the treatments had suddenly stopped working and her disease had progressed to the point where one foot was showing signs of gangrene. He sat before me, near despair, believing that he had lost his ability to heal. He had even begun to refer his patients to other therapists. I told him that he was not the problem, but that he should still stop treating her. Then I told him to bring his wife into my office, and I would explain what had happened later.

When his wife came in for an examination, I saw that her disease had indeed progressed to a dangerous point. My associate told me his diagnosis was excess fire energy in the lung channel—and I agreed. I then used my own energy, just as he had done, to give her a seemingly similar treatment. But within a few days her condition began to improve. Now my associate really began to doubt himself—until I explained what had happened.

He and his wife had been married for more than fifty years and continued to enjoy a very close, happy marriage. Just as some electricity moves in an alternating current, any kind of energy, even our own, needs an "opposite pole" to move to. What happened to my associate, simply put, was that after fifty years of marriage, the balance of his energy system was too similar to his wife's. Since her energy no longer represented an opposite pole, his energy could not interact with hers in the same way it used to—because they had become too similar. It's like the common observation that after many years of marriage couples even begin to look alike. At any rate, after a few more weeks of treatment, her diabetes was back under control. She continued to see me as a patient, with both her health and her husband's confidence restored.

Case Study # V

About ten years ago, Alan, a twenty-nine-year-old man suffering from testicular cancer, became my patient. During exploratory surgery a malignant tumor had been found in one of his testicles, and it had been removed. A blood test later showed that the cancer had begun to spread to his lymph system—a very dangerous sign. He was currently undergoing chemotherapy and was suffering from fatigue and hair loss. Having read about alternate cancer therapies, he came to me to discuss scaling back his chemotherapy. He said the treatments were his "security blanket"; but he felt he wanted to control his disease with natural methods that wouldn't leave him with stressful side effects. Our first step was to begin talking about his life before he came down with the cancer.

Alan was a successful executive in the music industry. But with that success came an extremely stressful lifestyle, with lots of smoking and drinking and little sleep. His diet consisted of cheeseburgers and french fries, and he lived in fear of losing his job. Unfortunately, he lost his health instead. The disease was telling him that his life was extremely out of balance. It told him his life had to change, and that he had to make his health a top priority.

Alan was living on disability benefits when we met, and these were about to run out. As he continued the chemotherapy, he came in regularly for acupuncture treatments to help alleviate the fatigue. He then began a new, less stressful career as a freelance writer covering the music industry. Next we changed his diet. The cheeseburgers and french fries were replaced with chicken and fish, fresh vegetables, whole grain breads and yogurt.

Alan had always been the person everybody else relied upon emotionally. Now he began counseling to learn how to take care of his own emotions first. He also began to study tai chi chuan, and practiced for an hour a day. We rounded out his new health plan by adding a cancer-fighting herbal therapy.

Within a few months he felt well enough and confident enough to stop chemotherapy. He continued taking good care of himself, and saw me regularly for both acupuncture and Q.M. therapy treatments to keep his energy system strong. Although he also continued going for blood tests every six months, within weeks there was no trace of the cancer. And today, ten years later, Alan remains in good health, requiring only an occasional treatment.

Case Study #VI

Every patient's case is different—even if they seem to be suffering from "common" illnesses. An illness may have one name so that we can identify it—a name based on how it manifests itself in the body—but the underlying patterns of disharmony can differ greatly, and must be treated accordingly.

At one point in my practice, I was simultaneously treating three different couples for infertility. Each couple came to me after exhausting all other treatments. No one could determine why either the couples were not able to conceive, or the women were not able to carry a child to term.

∞

Larry and Sara were a young couple, both in their early thirties, both in good general health. Yet Sara had been trying to conceive a child for more than four years without success, and no one had been able to determine why. Larry's sperm count seemed a little low, but well within what is considered normal. After taking Sara's pulses and examining her tongue, I determined that her overall energy was unusually balanced and strong—she was in terrific health.

Then I examined Larry. Right away I knew he was the problem. There was excess fire energy in both the liver and kidney channels. This "heat" was spilling over into the entire energy system—that is, his entire system was too hot and needed to be cooled down. The heat was due to an overall problem of congested energy—the energy was simply not flowing properly throughout his body. All this excess heat was affecting his sperm. Even though his sperm count was considered normal, the excess heat kept the count on the low side and negatively affected the way the sperm functioned.

Larry began to see me twice a month for acupuncture, Q.M. therapy, and herbal treatments, which all worked together to cool down his system. One-and-a-half years later Sara had a perfectly healthy baby boy.

∞

A second couple, Dan and Christine, both in their early forties, came to see me after having suffered through two miscarriages in the previous two years. It seemed that Christine, who was forty-two at the time, just wasn't able to bring a child to term. Dan checked out fine. After examining Christine, I found that she suffered from deficient energy in the kidney channel, which most likely was affecting the conception vessel, the energy channel associated with the uterus.

I found her problem had two basic underlying patterns of disharmony. The first was associated with the fact that she had delayed having a child for so long. When some women's reproductive cycle has continued operating in the same way for more than 40 years without conceiving, her body will eventually accept that to be "normal," and her energy will naturally strive to continue to flow in that way. So after all this time, when Christine tried to alter such a well-established pattern, her body's energy system tried to continue what it thought was normal functioning, which unfortunately resulted in two miscarriages.

The second pattern of disharmony concerned the weak energy in her conception vessel. Because energy precedes physical organs, her weak energy had weakened the structure of the uterus itself. After one year of treatment involving herbs, acupuncture, and Q.M. therapy, all aimed at altering these two patterns of disharmony, Christine gave birth to a healthy baby girl.

∞

Sam and Denise's case had me stumped at first. Both were in their late twenties and in good general health, yet Denise had been unable to become pregnant after three years of trying. After examining them both, the only clue I could find to their mysterious situation was that Denise had slightly deficient energy in her kidney channel. Other than that, nothing seemed to be wrong. They had already exhausted all types of infertility treatments before coming to me. So I started each of them on an "energy build-up" program involving herbs, acupuncture, and Q.M. therapy, to further strengthen their systems. Nothing worked.

Finally, Denise told me she had decided to give up her dream of having a family. I noticed she seemed somewhat relieved. I asked her if she was ambivalent about having a baby. She admitted she was slightly nervous. But as we continued to discuss it, I realized she wasn't just slightly nervous—she was *terrified* of the responsibility. I finally realized why Denise wasn't getting pregnant: Despite all her efforts, she really didn't want to. Her body was just following her mind's orders. I suggested she and Sam try some counseling to see if that would help. After taking my advice, they appeared back in my office a few weeks later. This time Denise told me she was afraid of becoming a mother but also wanted to face her fear and overcome it. Instead of infertility, I began to treat her for anxiety using acupuncture points in the ear. Three months later she became pregnant. Today, Sam and Denise are the proud parents of a baby girl.

∞

There is one important thing all of these cases have in common. All of the patients were fully committed to solving their health problems; they all were committed to getting better. This may seem like a somewhat obvious comment to make. Doesn't everyone want to get

better? The answer is no. Western culture actually re-
wards illness. We *use* illness to get out of things we
don't want to do or situations or emotions we don't
want to deal with. We also get a lot of attention when
we're sick: People visit us, give us flowers, and so on.
Every patient has to make a decision to get well and find
the courage to do the work to achieve good health. In
each of these cases, the patient continued to come to me
for treatment until he or she was completely cured.
Sometimes, when patients start to realize they are getting well, they actually stop coming for treatment. It
takes courage to change, and changing the state of your
health means you must change the entire state of your
being. This often involves doing some difficult emotional work that can be painful at times. Some people
are unwilling or unable to do this. And whenever one
person changes, the people around him often have to
change too. The emotional balance of marriages, fami-
lies, and even work relationships can all be called into
question—and all may have to change to accommodate
the new, healthy individual.

The road to health begins with recognizing that you
have a problem. Many people are not in touch with our
emotions; they literally have no idea what they are
feeling inside. Unresolved emotional conflicts are like
energy time bombs. When they go off, physical illness
often occurs. Check to see if you are really in touch
with your emotions. Read over some of the physical
ailments associated with the primary energy channels
and emotions. They may give you a clue to your state of
total well-being even if you are not consciously aware of
your life being out of balance. In order to make the most

of your own inner energy, to fully realize it, you need to determine the strengths and weaknesses of your unique system. I hope this chapter has helped you achieve some insight into yourself, and will help you change for the better—or perhaps just begin to realize that you need to change.

Not everyone needs to consult an energetic therapist. If you enjoy good general health but still want to feel even better—to boost your energy system—much of this work can be accomplished on your own. I recommend keeping a daily journal to help you find the patterns of disharmony within your own life. Keep track of all your physical symptoms and emotions, and your diet, weight, amount and type of exercise, the weather that day, stressful situations—everything and anything you can think of to write down. After a few months, you will start to find patterns in your life. You may find that you react to stressful situations by eating more sugar than you normally do, or that hot weather makes you irritable, or that a certain relationship is more important to your happiness than you realized. Start to make the connections and you will start to see what works in your life—and what needs to change, to be rebalanced.

While not everyone wants to change his or her life, almost everyone wants his or her life to be better. Even if the desired change seems minor, any change in your life will require a substantial amount of work. And only you have the power to change your own life. Your energy, the power within you, is completely under your control. And the key to controlling your life is to develop and control your powers of mental concentration through meditation. This is the ultimate key to your health and happiness. At the heart of all self-change is a redirection of mental energy—a change in the way you think. Whether emotional or physical healing is needed, all physicians, even energetic therapists, are just catalysts in the healing process. It is always your energy alone that does the actual healing. And it is always your *mind* that directs this energy and controls the healing process.

Develop your ability to see yourself changing. Give yourself permission to be whatever it is you want to be. Don't blame anybody or anything else for holding you back. You and you alone have the power to choose whether to change or to remain the same. Picture yourself doing the things you really want to do, reprogram your mind, and eventually you will become the person you see yourself becoming.

Using only your mind, you can not only heal your body, but change your entire life as well. Using only your ability to concentrate, you can engage your body's energy system and direct the energy *exactly* where you want it to go. You can have complete control over yourself, but in order to exercise this control you must increase your ability to concentrate. Changing your life, improving it, all starts with concentration and the ability to let your energy flow with your body. Once you master this, you will be able to let your entire being flow with the energies around you. In the next chapter I will show you how a balanced energetic diet and lifestyle will help you increase your inner energies. I guarantee that if you follow these simple guidelines, your life will improve. Life is a complicated balancing act, but in that balance lies your health and happiness. And once you take control of the power of your own energy, both health and happiness can be yours.

Chapter Five

MAXIMUM ENERGY FOR LIFE

A LIFE FILLED with maximum energy can only arise from an energetically balanced lifestyle. Your energy system is only completely balanced when all your energy is working for you, and none of it is being wasted. Long-term health and happiness will only be secured when your *entire* life is in balance. Internal energy imbalances are generally the result of an unbalanced lifestyle. In fact, it is impossible to separate an internal energy imbalance from an external lifestyle imbalance—or even determine which came first. And while it is true that all energy systems are basically alike when balanced, how and why they become unbalanced varies greatly from person to person.

This is why energetics avoids "blanket" remedies. For example, it is taken for granted in the West that aspirin is great medicine for headaches—and for most people this is true. But it is not true for everyone. Aspirin can make some people quite ill. Similarly, there are no simple blanket energy-balancing remedies that work for everyone. In order to balance your life energy—that is, balance your life—you have to *think for yourself.* This is much more troublesome then following specific health guidelines that supposedly work for everyone. It takes constant work. You have to get in touch with the energy that runs throughout both your body and your mind—and *listen* to it. Your energy system is unique. It knows what it needs for both physical and emotional health. From eating right to getting the right amount of sleep, there are no rigid rules to follow, no blanket remedies; you alone can learn what's right for you.

Overall, an energetically balanced lifestyle is based on simple common sense. This means doing everything in moderation. So in order to balance your life energy, you have to rebalance the *way* you think and live. Apply the concept of *yin* and *yang* to every aspect of your life. Just as daytime coexists in balance with nighttime, so does activity with sleep, diet with exercise, and so on. Any illness, including being overtired or overweight, is a sign that your life is not in balance. While some of these signs may not seem serious to you now, they could, if left uncorrected over a long period of time, have very serious consequences.

Unfortunately, serious illness is often what it takes to finally "wake people up" to the fact that their lives are out of balance. Don't let this happen to you. Begin to examine the balance of your entire life now. In my practice, I see the same four underlying reasons why my patients' energy systems have become unbalanced: an inability to get in touch with and balance their emotions, improper sleeping habits, a lack of proper exercise, and an improper diet. When I use the term "improper," I mean they are not doing what is right for them. I find myself prescribing the following four-point "balancing system" over and over again:

1. Begin a Program of Daily Meditation that's Right for You. People's health and overall well-being become seriously unbalanced when small signs of imbalance are ignored over a long period of time. As the gap widens between the proper amount and type of energy that our systems need and what we are actually receiving, serious and sometimes irreversible illness can result. Large imbalances are much more difficult to correct than small ones. With proper, continual care and attention, minor energy imbalances can be completely or substantially corrected. This means you must think about your energy, both emotional and physical, and get in touch with it through meditation *every day*. Put aside at least fifteen minutes for quiet time that is yours alone. Different methods work best for different people. Find whatever works best for you, whether it's following a structured TM program or just listening to music by yourself, and do it on a regular, daily basis.

Balanced lives begin with balanced decision-making. With all the distractions of our complex lives, making balanced decisions has probably never been more difficult. As you saw in the previous chapter, simply by concentrating your mental energy, you can balance both your mind's energy and your body's energy. Balanced mental energy leads to balanced thinking; balanced thinking leads to balanced decision-making; and balanced decision-making leads to a balanced life.

2. Start Exercising. Many of my patients' energy imbalances are due to or exacerbated by insufficient exercise. The amount of energy they take in as food exceeds the amount of energy expended as physical activity. The resulting excess energy is stored as fat and usually leads to a variety of internal energy imbalances. Exercise must always be balanced with diet. It's simple: The more you eat the more you should exercise in order to maintain your weight. If you need to lose weight, eat less and exercise more. If you need to gain weight, eat more and exercise less. But in either case, just as you *have* to eat to maintain your level of energy, you also *have* to exercise. It is not a choice. It is a necessity for a balanced life.

The importance of exercise in a balanced life goes beyond just maintaining your weight. Some people with naturally high metabolisms seem to be able to eat whatever and however much they want without exercising—without gaining an ounce. But this doesn't mean they don't have to exercise. Because exercise engages both mental and physical energy simultaneously, it also balances mind and body energy. It is one of the most powerful antistress remedies we have available to us. Most Westerners lead sedentary lives, which means we use more mental than physical energy. This creates an energy imbalance that can only be corrected by a proper exercise program.

Determining the right way for you to exercise begins with understanding what exercise is. As I discussed in chapter 1, when most Westerners think about their own "energy" they think about physical activity: moving around, getting things done. This same limited thinking is applied to exercise. Exercise is anything that gets your energy moving. Tennis, jogging, and aerobics are just three forms of exercise where activating your body activates your energy system. If you enjoy participating in these types of exercise, good—keep doing them. But if you don't, there is another way to get your energy moving.

As you know from previous chapters, you do not have to necessarily move around physically in order to move your energy. I find the reason many of my patients don't exercise is because they don't enjoy it. And while tennis and jogging are enjoyable and beneficial to some people, to others they could be too stressful, or even physically impossible. So when you need to exercise right, you need to find the right kind of exercise for you: the kind you will really do.

For people who hate to exercise in the Western sense of the word, or for those who suffer from illnesses like arthritis which prevent them from exercising, I have designed an energetic program comprised of different Q.M. exercises. This program, presented in the next chapter, is based on simple exercises similar to those that comprise tai chi chuan, yoga, and the martial arts. Even though they are not physically taxing, these exercises fully engage and balance the energy system, increase muscle tone, and provide all the same health benefits as vigorous Western exercises do. In addition, they are simple to learn, easy to do, and can be done in the privacy of your home, in the office, anywhere and anytime.

Once you find the right kind of exercise for you, make sure you incorporate it into your life properly. Whenever you begin to rebalance your life energy, you *must* do it gradually. If you have never exercised, suddenly embarking on an overly ambitious exercise program could do you more damage than good. *Never shock your energy system.* If you want to start playing tennis, jogging, or taking aerobics classes, always begin with at least ten minutes of stretching. Then begin slowly. Start with just a few minutes of exercise and gradually increase the amount and intensity over a period of three or four weeks. Again, there are no rigid rules. It is important to begin gradually and work toward a level of exercise you can regularly maintain. The same holds true if you used to exercise regularly and then suddenly stopped. You must gradually work up to speed all over again. You cannot stop exercising for weeks and then vigorously work out one day for three hours in an effort to "make up" the time you missed. This is too shocking to your energy system, and may radically unbalance it. Remember, it is better for your energy system to exercise each day for only ten minutes than to suddenly exercise intensely for a few hours a few times a month.

3. Get the Right Amount of Sleep. Getting too little or too much sleep can be extremely draining to your energy. Although many people do best with seven or eight hours per night, this is not true for everyone. Again, you have to listen to your body. If you do not feel rested even though you feel you have gotten the proper amount of sleep, this means you are not attaining the proper level of rest you need for your body to repair itself. Just as one type of energy sustains your activity throughout the day, another type sustains the proper level of rest at night. When these energies are out of balance, the result is chronic fatigue.

If you feel you are getting too little sleep, this may be because your "active" energy is out of balance. This means that either your active mind energy or your active body energy is working too hard. This will deplete the "rest" energy that sustains the proper level of undisturbed sleep your body needs. Conversely, if your active energy is not working hard enough, if not enough energy is expended during the day through mental or physical activity, this will give rise to too much "rest" energy, and you will sleep longer than you actually need to. Sleeping too much is another example of how "more is less." The healing powers of sleep are only effective when they are balanced. Too much sleep is draining to your energy, and is often a symptom of depression. When you work up to and maintain your proper level of exercise, your energy will naturally balance itself out. Insomnia and depression will often "automatically" disappear.

4. Eat an Energetically Balanced Diet. A good diet is more about what you should eat than what you shouldn't. Eating a proper diet means understanding what you need to eat, and when. A balanced diet is one that is balanced with the rest of your life. The Western concept of a balanced diet is one that includes the "right" amount of protein, carbohydrates, fat, and fiber—one that is supposedly "right" for everyone. This seems like sound advice, except that it ignores two important facts: Nothing is "right" for everyone, and different foods contain *different types of energy*. In other words, energetically speaking, all protein is not created equal. The same holds true for carbohydrates and fats. In order to understand an energetically balanced diet, we need to refer back to the five phases of energy (see table 5). These five different types of energy have been found to be contained within food, just as they are found within everything else that is part of our world.

Western science breaks things down in an effort to understand them, and it treats food in a similar way. But it is not enough to break foods down into their basic components. Again, Western science ignores the energetic properties of the world around us. According to Western theory, a balanced diet could include eating the proper amounts of, say, chicken, sweet potatoes, and salad, with peaches and strawberries for desert, every day. But according to energetics, eating this way over time might lead to a serious energy imbalance. That's because most of these foods contain "warm" energy. And consuming too many foods that contain a similar type of energy can, and most likely will, unbalance a person's energy system. In order to understand the different energetic natures of different foods, it is first helpful to understand how they are determined.

Table 5

PHASE:	Wood	Fire	Earth	Metal	Water
SEASON:	Spring	Summer	Late summer	Autumn	Winter
FOOD ENERGY:	Warm	Hot	Neutral	Cool	Cold

Determining the energetic nature of anything is a very complicated task, and a full discussion of the ancient and modern methods of doing so is beyond the scope of this book. But basically, it is accomplished through intense observation. Ancient scientists in the East first began studying medicinal herbs in their natural states to obtain clues to the essence of their energy. They recorded which season the herbs grew in, and whether they grew upward toward the sky or downward into the earth; they noted the color, scent, and so on. Over thousands of years, they began to understand the association between herbs and different types of energy—and how the energy of these herbs could powerfully affect human energy systems and health.

Herbology is an important part of energetic medicine. I often prescribe herbs in my own practice, always warning my patients not to use them indiscriminately. Just as you wouldn't walk behind the counter of your local pharmacy and help yourself to whatever prescriptive medicines you could find, I strongly advise you not to walk into a health food store and buy herbs without consulting a professional holistic health practitioner first. Herbal teas are usually fine for the general public, but taking a substantial amount of the wrong type of herb could actually be quite dangerous to your health. Remember that many Western medications that can only be obtained through a doctor's prescription are based on the same herbs that are available to you over the counter in many health food stores—so be careful.

As herbs were intensely studied in an effort to determine their energetic properties, so, too, were different animals, fruits, vegetables, and byproducts that became a part of the Oriental diet. The energetic nature of food is determined by how foods make us feel, how they interact with our energy systems. For example, coffee contains warm energy. This is true for both hot coffee and iced coffee, because it has to do with the type of energy within the coffee bean itself. The effect of a food's temperature on your energy system is short-lived. Within minutes your body will naturally cool down the hot coffee or heat up the iced coffee to 98.6 degrees, its internal temperature, so that the coffee can be easily assimilated into the body's energy system. But once that is accomplished, the coffee's warm energy will be extracted from the coffee itself. And this warm energy will actually "warm up" your energy system.

While the temperature of food does have some effect on the body's energy system (which we will discuss later), it ultimately has nothing to do with the food's energetic nature. Coffee, whether hot or iced, will warm your energy system. On the other hand, tea, which has a cool energy, will cool your system regardless of whether it is hot tea or iced tea. So if it is a very hot summer day and you want to cool down, it is actually better to drink a cup of hot tea than a glass of iced coffee.

In order to eat an energetically balanced diet, you need to eat a variety of foods with different energies. Luckily, this follows common sense. Most people would quickly get tired of eating chicken every day. Still, many popular diets over the years have advised just that: They have recommended that, in order to lose weight, one should eat the same food or foods every day for an extended period of time. This kind of unbalanced approach to eating can be extremely dangerous.

Each meal should consist of a meat (or protein substitute), a vegetable, and a grain. But the energies contained within all three should be varied from meal to meal and day to day. When an energetic therapist designs a balanced energetic diet plan, all the needed proteins and vitamins will be naturally included without having to be measured—so you will be eating a balanced, nutritional diet, even from a Western nutritional point of view.

The lists of different "food energies" in this book are just general guidelines to help you understand the concept of balancing your food's energetic properties (see table 6). Unfortunately, these lists are somewhat limited. The energetic properties of most Eastern foods have been determined, but many of these are not eaten or even available in the West. Also, remember that the energies of foods frequently change when cooked. Cooking with wine, salt, and different spices, or frying in butter as opposed to peanut oil, affects a food's energetic nature. Still, these lists should prove helpful in understanding the variety of foods contained in an energetically balanced diet, and should help you begin to apply the basic principles of energetics to your daily life.

While the foods that comprise an energetically balanced diet contain a variety of different food energies, the *amount* of food consumed must also be in balance with the rest of your lifestyle. If you exercise or work vigorously every day, you should eat more than if you sit at a desk all day. Most Western diets, because of the wide variety of foods available relative to many others in the world, are actually quite balanced. The major dietary problem in the West is that we eat far too much. Even many of those who exercise do not exercise enough to balance out their food intake. Again, all one really needs to do is to use common sense. Listen to your body. Only eat when you are hungry and stop when you *feel* that you have had enough. This is certainly a simple idea, but how many of us actually follow it? Your body requires a certain amount of food to extract energy from. It tells you when it needs food, and how much food it needs. Learn to listen to it. Ignoring your body's requests or eating poor-quality food over a long period of time will lead to energy imbalances and illness.

The stomach energy channel is responsible for taking in the body's food, and the spleen channel works to extract the energy from the ingested food. When you eat too much, you are overwhelming your digestive energy system. You are forcing it to work too hard. Therefore, you are actually draining your own overall energy— which is why you feel so tired and sluggish after eating a large meal. When you continue to do this to your body over a long period of time, you are depleting the energy in your stomach and spleen channels, which can lead to energy imbalances in other channels—and to a variety of illnesses. Overweight people often suffer from fatigue not only because they have more weight to carry around, but also because their energy systems are chronically being drained and put out of balance. In addition, weight gain can decrease the sex drive, not only because of the psychological factors, but also because excess food intake leads to excess energy in the stomach channel. The body balances out this excess energy by lessening the energy in the kidney channel, the energy channel that governs an individual's sex drive.

FOODS WITH WARM ENERGY

Meat and Fish	Dairy Products
Anchovies	Butter
Beef	
Chicken	
Chicken liver	
Duck	
Lamb	
Mussels	
Pork	
Shrimp	

Fruits, Vegetables, and Legumes	Herbs and Spices
Brown sugar	Basil
Capers	Bay leaf
Cherries	Cinnamon
Chestnuts	Coriander
Chives	Dill seed
Cloves	Fennel seed
Coconut milk	Garlic
Coffee	Ginger
Dates	Ginseng
Leeks	Nutmeg
Litchi nuts	Rosemary
Mustard greens	Spearmint

Fruits, Vegetables, and Legumes	Herbs and Spices
Onions	
Peaches	
Pine nuts	
Safflower	
Scallions	
Squash	
Strawberries	
Sweet potatoes	
Vinegar	
Walnuts	

FOODS WITH HOT ENERGY

Meat and Fish	Herbs and Spices
Trout	Black pepper
	Cayenne pepper
	Cinnamon
	Ginger (dried)

Fruits, Vegetables, and Legumes	
Green peppers	

FOODS WITH NEUTRAL ENERGY

Meat and Fish	Dairy Products
Eggs	Cheese
Herring	Milk
Mako shark	
Oysters	
Sardines	
Sturgeon	
Tuna fish	
White fish	

Fruits, Vegetables, and Legumes		Herbs and Spices
Almonds	Peanuts	Saffron
Apricots	Peanut oil	
Beets	Peas	
Cabbage	Pineapple	
Carrots	Plums	
Celery	Potatoes	
Coconut	Pumpkin	
Corn	Raspberries	
Figs	Rice	
Grapes	Rye	
Honey	Shiitake mushrooms	
Kidney beans	String beans	
Olives	Sugar	
Papaya	Turnips	
	Yams	

FOODS WITH COOL ENERGY

Fruits, Vegetables, and Legumes	Herbs and Spices
Apples	Marjoram
Barley	Peppermint
Celery	
Cucumber	
Eggplant	
Gluten	
Lettuce (except romaine)	
Millet	
Mushrooms	
Pears	
Radishes	

FOODS WITH COOL ENERGY (*Continued*)

Fruits, Vegetables, and Legumes	*Herbs and Spices*
Sesame oil	
Spinach	
Swiss chard	
Tea	
Tofu	
Watercress	
Wheat	
Wheat bran	

FOODS WITH COLD ENERGY

Meat and Fish	*Herbs and Spices*
Clams	Salt
Crabs	White pepper
Octopus	

Fruits, Vegetables, and Legumes
Asparagus
Bamboo shoots
Bananas
Grapefruit
Kelp
Mangos
Mulberries
Musk melons
Oranges
Persimmons
Plantains
Romaine lettuce

Fruits, Vegetables, and
  Legumes

Seaweed
Tomatoes
Water chestnuts
Watermelon
Wheat germ

But there are still other ways many of us overtax our digestive energy. Our internal temperature naturally remains at approximately 98.6 degrees. When you eat food that is overly hot or overly cold (in terms of temperature), the stomach energy channel has to work harder to cool it down or heat it up so that it can be digested. This takes energy. In addition, raw foods are harder for your body to break down than cooked foods; eating too many fruits, vegetables, and nuts can actually deplete your digestive energy.

Food is an important part of any culture. And here lie great differences between the East and West. In the East, food is prepared and chosen like medicine. You eat what is good for you more than what you may like to eat. Oftentimes, when ordering a meal in an Eastern restaurant, you do so by describing how you feel that day, or your symptoms if you are ill. In the West, food is more often associated with pleasure; you eat simply what *tastes* good to you, whether it is good for you or not. This is why so many Westerners eat too many sweets: They taste good to most people. But too much sugar depletes stomach and spleen energy, another reason for the Western population's continual battle against weight gain.

When attempting to lose weight, it is also bad to follow diets that "clean you out"—like suddenly fasting for a few days, or drinking only water or herbal teas. Such practices are not good for you, and this kind of unbalanced thinking will upset the balance of your internal energy. We are not machines that get dirty and need to be "cleaned out" periodically. Eat sensibly and you will find a diet that you can really live with, without any need for crash diets or fasting. Adopting an energetically balanced diet will naturally help you lose weight and keep it off.

An energetically balanced life also maintains a healthy balance between our internal energy and the external energies around us. Therefore, a balanced energetic diet changes with the seasons. In order to be in harmony with the energy of the universe, you should eat foods that are in balance with the energy of the current season. Always move in harmony with the seasons, changing your diet as the world changes around you. When it is hot outside you naturally want to "balance it out" by eating foods that will cool your internal energy, like tuna fish and salads. In wintertime, you naturally want to eat more meats or other foods that contain warm energy. Continually readjusting the balance of your diet by complementing the energies of the seasons will keep your energy in balance, and so at its peak level all year long. This basic concept assumes that a person's energy is reasonably balanced. If this is not the case, common sense again redefines what should be eaten.

Only after an extensive examination can an energetic therapist determine how and why your energy system is out of balance, and then prescribe a proper diet for you. And determining a patient's proper diet can only be accomplished after determining the state of the person's basic energetic constitution. This, of course, can be extremely complicated. The following exercise is just to show you how the process works in general:

Most people have one of two basic physical constitutions: hot or cold. People who have a "hot" energetic constitution often feel hot and thirsty. Their hands and feet tend to be hot and sweaty; they prefer cold drinks, and often have tongues that are deep red. People with "cold" constitutions often have cold hands and feet, generally prefer hot drinks to cold drinks, and have tongues that are more pale in color. Most people have mixed constitutions, so prescribing dietary therapy is rarely easy. The general rules, however, are quite simple. People with overly hot energy should eat more foods from the cool and cold energy categories *throughout the year*; and rarely eat those foods with hot and warm energies—or, in some cases, avoid them completely. This is because even though it may be extremely cold outside, these peoples' energy systems may still be "too hot" inside, resulting in an internal/external energy imbalance—too wide a gap between hot and cold. Despite the cold environment, their internal energies still may have to be cooled down. The same idea would be applied to people with cold constitutions. They should eat more hot and warm energy foods throughout the year, and avoid those with cool and cold energy. In addition, the symptoms of imbalance will worsen in corresponding weather. So a hot person's symptoms will worsen in hot weather and a cold person's in cold weather. Maintaining a proper balance can become even more complicated, because a cold person could have a hot illness, or vice versa. So balanced diets must be continually readjusted according to common sense after all energetic factors (regarding both internal and external energy) are taken into account. At least one thing that is easy to remember is that foods with "neutral" energy are already balanced, and so may be eaten in moderation by almost everyone all year long.

An energetically balanced diet is not just an important part of maintaining a balanced energy system and preventing illness; it is also an important element in rebalancing energy, in *curing* illnesses. Dietary therapy is usually a supplement to other energetic treatments, but often plays an important role. Specific foods act on specific energy channels in different ways. Once the food you eat is transformed into energy within your body, it unites with the body's energy in different channels. From here it moves within your body in different ways. The energy from some foods moves upward, downward, outward, or inward, and can counteract an incorrect flow of energy.

To understand this phenomenon, think of the body as being divided into four different regions: above the waist, below the waist, the internal region, and the exterior region or skin surface. Some foods—like wine, for instance—cause the body's energy to move upward, and can be used to counteract illnesses caused by too much energy moving downward. That's why a little wine will help alleviate circulatory problems, increasing the upward flow of blood (and also why drinking too much wine can cause dizziness and a red face). On the other hand, salt causes the body's energy to move downward, part of the reason why people who experience swelling in the lower part of the body need to regulate the amount of salt they use. Foods like ginger move energy outward and lower fevers by inducing perspiration. And foods that move energy inward, like sugar, tend to aid in digestion. Many foods also contain two different energies that move in different directions. An energetic therapist must, of course, take all of these considerations into account before recommending a diet that will balance out your unique energy system.

Both the causes and cures of different allergies are continually debated in Western science. In energetics medicine, allergies are explained in terms of severe energy imbalances. For example, walnuts are among the foods that increase the energy in the kidney channel; so if a patient who already suffers from a severe excess of energy in this channel eats some walnuts, the energy system may react in a variety of ways, including a sudden asthmatic attack. In terms of energetics, an allergic reaction occurs when the energy system "rejects" a sudden supply of energy it can't handle, because that supply suddenly worsens an existing energy imbalance to the point where it poses a dangerous threat to the overall system. In this instance, if the initial energy imbalance in the kidney channel were corrected, the patient would be able to eat walnuts without any reaction.

Because some foods affect the flow of energy in specific channels, and the flow of energy in specific channels both creates and is created by certain emotions, there exists a direct relationship between foods and emotions. An energetically balanced diet can help you control your moods—or even create them. Depression is often created by a lack of energy. Foods like garlic and ginger often work as natural anti-depressants, because they increase energy throughout the system. People naturally reach for different foods to rebalance themselves when they are angry, happy, or anxious, often without any conscious awareness of doing so.

There are many popular misconceptions about which foods are good for us and which are bad. It is not true that sugar, salt, red meat, milk, and "deadly nightshade" vegetables like potatoes, onions, and tomatoes are all bad for all of us. In general, they are all fine if consumed in moderation. For most of us sugar and salt, consumed in moderation, are okay to eat, and for some people, they form a necessary part of the diet. A little sugar aids digestion and a little salt helps regulate bodily fluids. The problem with sugar and salt is that most Americans consume much too much of them. From our breakfast cereals to ketchup, sugar and salt are hidden in more foods than most of us know. And how many of us add salt to our food before even tasting it? The same holds true for red meat, milk, and the "deadly nightshade" vegetables. All are fine for most people if eaten *in moderation* like everything else.

But there are certain foods and substances that deplete energy, even when consumed in moderation:

- Fried foods;
- Foods barbecued over charcoal, especially charred meats;
- Coffee, *including* decaffeinated coffee;

- Alcohol (except when used in cooking where it is burned off); and
- Cigarettes, pipes, or cigars.

Diet is another powerful energy tool that is under your complete control—a tool you can use every day to increase and control your own energy. An energetically balanced diet can prevent an energy imbalance before it occurs or help to rebalance your system. When designing your own energetically balanced diet, always eat a variety of fresh seasonal foods that will "balance out" your internal energy, always eat and drink in moderation, avoid too many raw foods or those that are overly hot or overly cold, and try to stay away from energy-depleting foods and habits as much as possible.

Energetics is a realistic approach to life. Its concepts work for everyone because it accepts the fact that *each of us is unique.* Everyone must find his or her own balance; and there are no rigid rules that apply to everyone on how to get there. Following the guidelines in this book will help you begin to live a balanced life filled with maximum energy. And you should start realizing results within only a few weeks.

Life is stressful because it is constantly changing. Energetics can help you cope with stress by helping you learn to naturally rebalance yourself, no matter what changes are occurring in the outside world. Physical and emotional health are always the result of balanced internal energy. Diseases are not simply "caught" from other people or from the outside world; one way or another, they always start inside us, as an energy imbalance that allows them to enter and further disrupt our energy system. Keeping your energy balanced will help you develop the inner strength you need to stay healthy in an increasingly stressful world.

Always remember that the secret to a life filled with health and happiness, a life filled with maximum energy, isn't necessarily exercising more, eating more, sleeping more, or doing more of anything—it is keeping these things ever in balance.

Chapter Six

THIRTY MINUTES, THIRTY DAYS TO MAXIMUM ENERGY

MAXIMUM ENERGY comes from balanced energy. And balanced energy comes from a balanced life. But when your life is out of balance, how do you realign it? Where do you begin? The thirty-day energetic workout can help you get started. This structured exercise program is designed to help you gradually balance both your body energy and your mind energy. When your mind and body energy are in balance, you will not only look and feel better, but also start making better decisions about your entire life. As you undertake the enormous task of rebalancing your life, it is important to proceed on all fronts, but the thirty-day energetic workout is a good place to start.

Energetic exercises combine mental concentration with physical and breathing exercises, harmonizing mind, body, and universal energies. Practiced for thousands of years, these exercises draw on some of the basic movements common to Eastern exercise programs like yoga, tai chi chuan, and the martial arts. Tai chi chuan and yoga are both ancient energy-balancing techniques that synchronize breathing with extremely focused, yet peaceful, mental concentration. Both have been shown to dramatically lower oxygen consumption, slow down metabolic activity, and calm the nervous system. Because they increase and harmonize energy flow, they have been found to be effective healers of many chronic conditions, including high blood pressure and depression. By combining mental concentration with correct posture, breathing, and movement, each exercise stimulates key energy centers just as acupuncture and other energetic therapies do. These simple exercises are deceptively powerful. When performed correctly, they increase the flow of energy and will, over time, naturally remove minor energy blockages and keep others from occurring.

But not everyone has the time or patience to study tai chi chuan and yoga. Tai chi chuan is a complicated twenty-minute exercise that can take up to five years to learn correctly. And many yoga positions require flexibility and balance which can also take years to achieve. The exercise program in this chapter works with the same principles as tai chi chuan and yoga do and is just as effective, but it takes only one month to learn.

There are thousands of energetic exercises that will increase and balance different areas of your energy system. I have designed this program around eight exercises I have found to be particularly effective. Performed together, these eight simple exercises will balance out all twelve major meridians and increase flexibility, muscle tone, and stamina. They are easy to learn and simple to do, and the entire program can easily be committed to memory. This way, no matter where you are, whether at home or at the office or even on the road, you can always work on increasing and balancing your energy.

The thirty-day energetic workout begins with understanding how important correct posture is—and *what* it is. Standing "at attention" with shoulders back, stomach in, and locked knees may be considered correct posture in the U.S. Army, but it is not good for your energy system. Standing in this rigid way causes muscles to tense. Tense muscles will not only keep your energy from flowing smoothly, they will also deplete your energy system because your body consumes more energy in getting these muscles to tighten and stay that way. Energetically correct posture is shown in photo 1. Feet should be placed shoulder-width apart, with weight evenly distributed. Eyes should look straight ahead, neither up nor down, while shoulders are relaxed and slightly rounded, arms hang naturally, buttocks are slightly tucked inward, and knees are slightly bent.

When you find a quiet, relaxed place to perform your energetic workout, begin by practicing this basic posture for two or three minutes at a time. When standing this way, use your mind to relax your body. Tell your body to relax. Feel the tension drain out from the bottoms of your feet and from the tips of your fingers. As your body relaxes, your mind will begin to relax as well. Concentrate on clearing your mind of thoughts and just allow yourself to *be*. After a few minutes you will feel your energy begin to balance itself out.

After you have practiced your energetic posture and can relax your body "at will," you can begin to work on proper breathing technique. After standing in the basic energetic posture for a few minutes and reaching an overall relaxed state, place your hands a few inches below your navel (see photo 2). As you slowly breathe in air through your nose, gently push your hands outward with your breath. As you exhale through your nose, feel your hands move in with your breath as well. Never hold your breath. Let your mind control your breathing. Continue to concentrate on your breathing until it be-

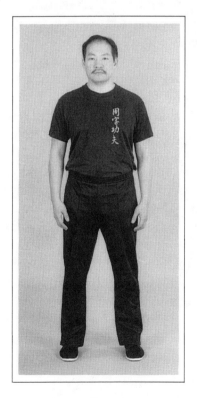
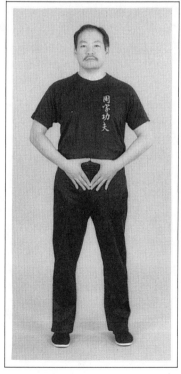

comes naturally effortless. Now take the tip of your tongue and gently rest it on the front of the roof of your mouth, swallowing saliva when you have to. This simple practice completes an important "energy circuit," and will help the energy circulate more easily and evenly throughout your entire system. Once you have mastered the energetic posture and breathing technique, you are ready to begin learning the thirty-day energetic workout.

The energetic workout begins with a five-minute stretching routine. A simple daily routine like this is a critical element in keeping your energy flowing and balanced. Stretching is the best exercise to do when you barely have the time to exercise at all. Just a few minutes a day is all you need to become and stay flexible. By freeing the joints and loosening tight muscles, stretching helps blocked energy flow freely throughout the body to where it is needed. It is the single most effective way to naturally keep yourself looking and feeling younger.

At first, just familiarize yourself with each stretch by performing them *once or twice only*. Do them as well as you *comfortably* can. Muscles have to be loosened gradually. Don't attempt the advanced stretches until you actually begin the thirty-day energetic workout. Each stretch should be performed *slowly*, in a relaxed manner and with no bouncing. Follow each instruction, and make sure you are breathing properly. When you actually begin the workout, the stretching warm-up should take approximately five minutes. If it is taking you less time, slow down—you are doing them too quickly.

Thirty-Day Energetic Work-out

Five-Minute Stretch

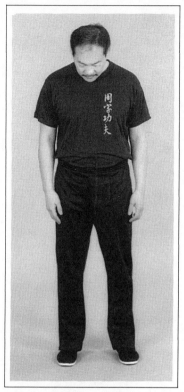

Stress often causes the muscles supporting the head to become tight, and this can lead to a variety of problems. That's why we begin with stretching these important muscles.

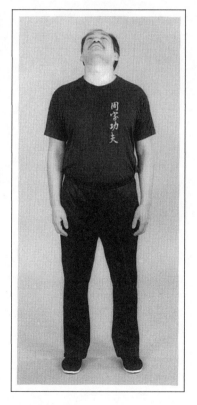

After finding your own natural stance, begin the five-minute stretch warm-up by slowly *bending your head forward as far as you comfortably can, and then slowly backward. Repeat each movement eight times.*

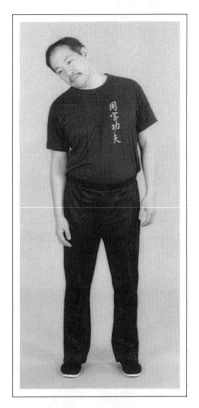

Keeping shoulders down, bend your head to the right, and then slowly rotate it backward to the left. After coming back to center, repeat to the left.

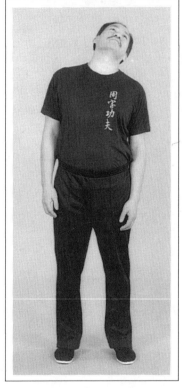

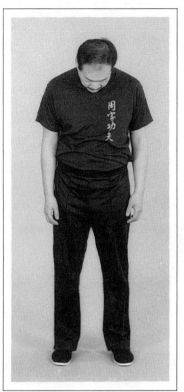

As you rotate your head, feel which muscles are tighter than the others to become aware of where you are retaining tension in your neck. Repeat three times in each direction.

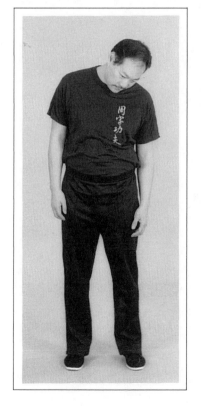

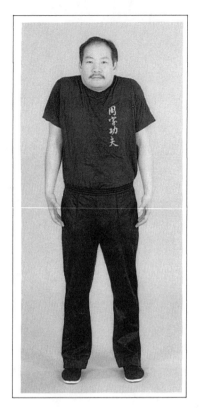

Shrug your shoulders as high as you comfortably can. Rotate your shoulders backward slowly, always coming back to the original position. Repeat eight times to the back and then eight times to the front.

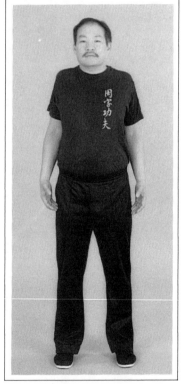

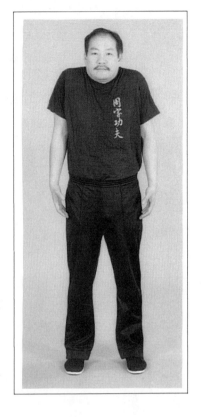

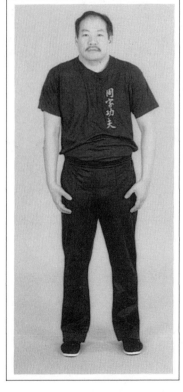

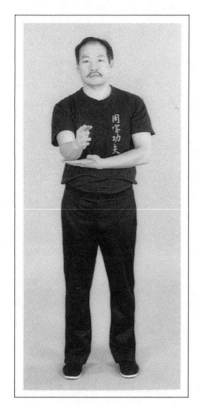

Supporting your right elbow with your left palm, rotate your right forearm to the right, simultaneously flexing your right wrist.

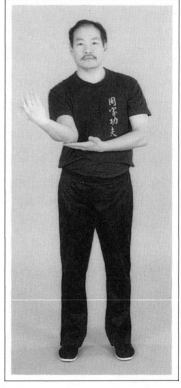

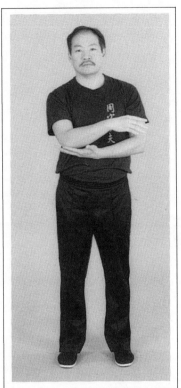

Repeat eight times in each direction. Change arms and repeat eight times in each direction again.

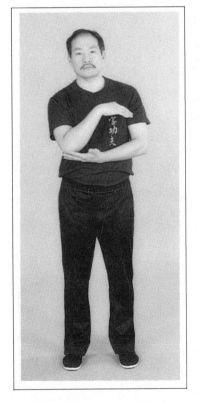

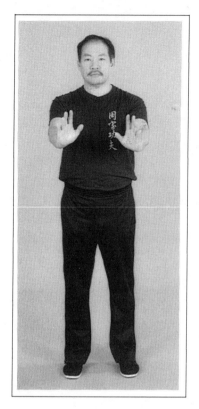

Extending both arms forward, rotate your wrists away from your body in a downward circular motion. Repeat eight times then reverse, rotating your wrists toward your body eight times.

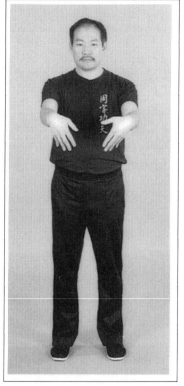

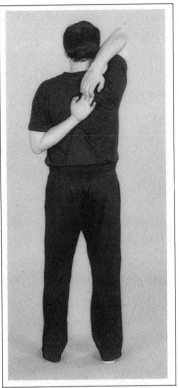

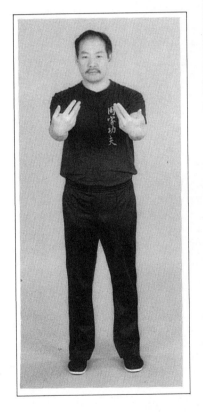

Loosen your arms and shoulders by touching hands behind your back as shown here. If you cannot do this easily, do as much as you can without straining (grasping a rolled up towel in your hands may help). Repeat three times alternately on each side.

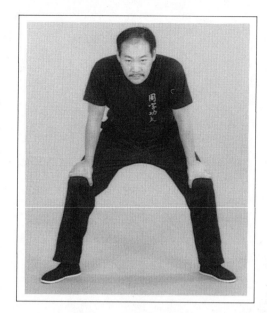

Spread your feet wider than shoulder-width apart. Lean forward with thumbs on the inside of each thigh over the knee.

Slowly lean to the right and hold for three seconds.

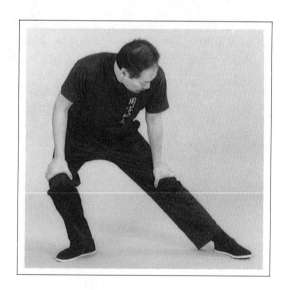

Transfer your weight to the left side and hold for three seconds. Repeat the movement eight times on each side.

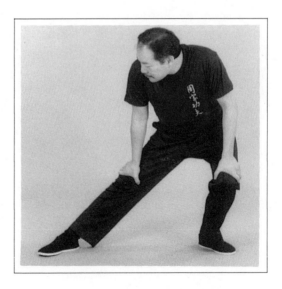

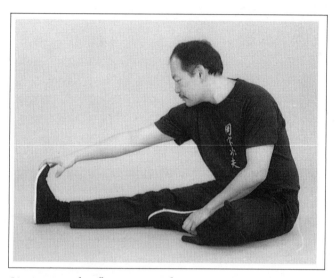

Sitting on the floor, extend your right leg forward with your left leg bent inward. Lean forward as much as possible (do not force beyond what feels comfortable) and hold for three seconds. Sit up, then repeat two more times. Change legs and repeat the stretch on left side.

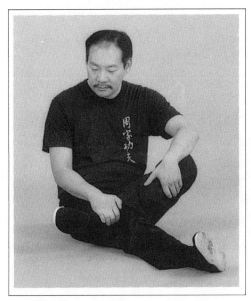

Crossing one leg over the other, slowly rotate your ankle forward and backward three times. Switch legs and repeat.

Advanced Stretches

(The three advanced stretches should add another minute to the stretch warm-up.)

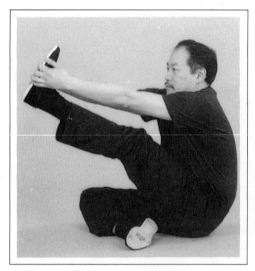

Still sitting, clasp both hands around the bottom of one foot. Slowly extend the leg as much as possible. Hold for three seconds and release. Repeat on other leg.

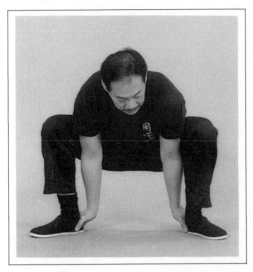

Starting with your hands behind your ankles, slowly straighten your legs as much as possible. Hold for three seconds. Return to the starting position and repeat eight times.

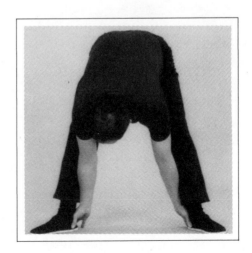

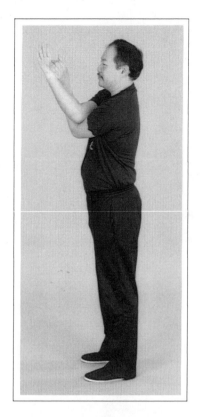

Intertwine your arms as shown and hold for five seconds. Reverse arms and repeat.

The second part of the thirty-day energetic workout contains the eight basic energetic exercises that will increase and balance your inner energy. By alternately relaxing and tensing muscles, combining slow movements with held positions, these exercises stretch and relax the muscles around certain organs. This increases the energy circulation around the organs and stimulates important energy centers. Next to the descriptions that accompany each exercise, I have shown the specific energy channels the exercise affects.

The program is designed to gradually increase your energy, not to shock your system. It gives you the time you need to learn each exercise and commit it to memory so that you can use all your mental concentration on performing the exercise without concentrating on the instructions. This way you will also gradually increase your powers of concentration. Mental concentration is critical to each exercise. As you try out each one, move slowly and focus on feeling the movement of your inner energy within your body. As your powers of concentration develop, you will be amazed at your ability to actually *feel* the energy moving within specific channels. Again, as you try out each exercise, do it *slowly*. Each exercise should take approximately three minutes to complete.

Exercises

1. Balances heart, liver, spleen, lung, and kidney channels.

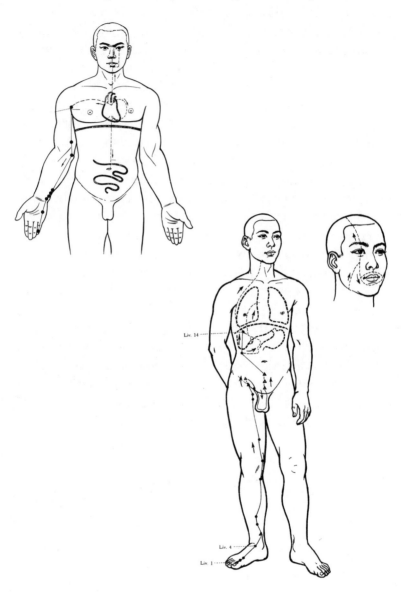

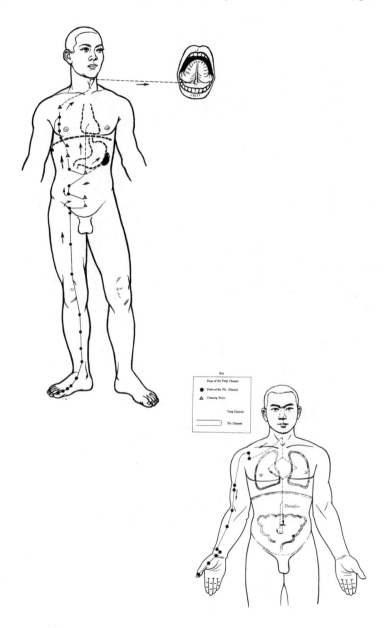

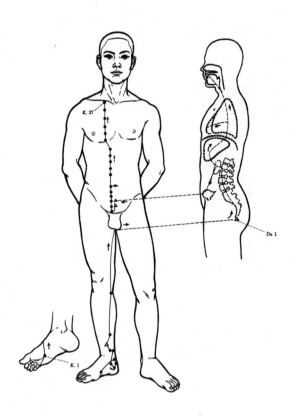

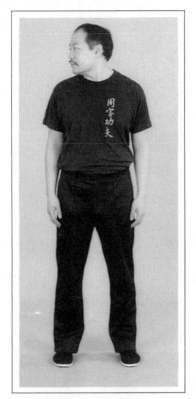

Begin with your body in a natural stance. Without moving the rest of your body, slowly turn your head to the right as far as you comfortably can to look over your shoulder.

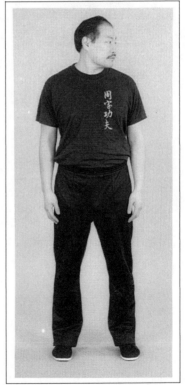

Return to the center and repeat to the left. Repeat the exercise eight times on each side.

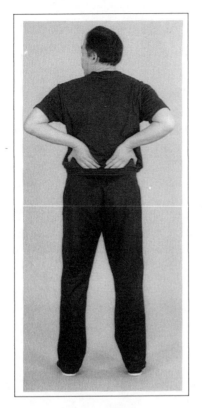

Place your hands on your back as shown. Holding this position, repeat looking over each shoulder, eight times on each side.

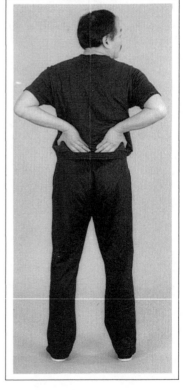

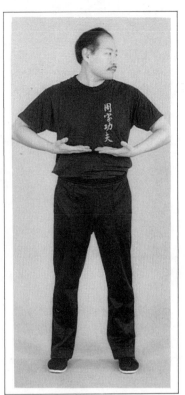

Change your hands to face inward, palms up, as shown. Hold this position as you repeat the exercise again, eight times on each side.

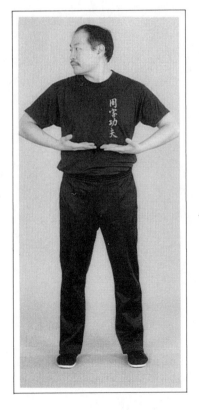

2. Balances all channels

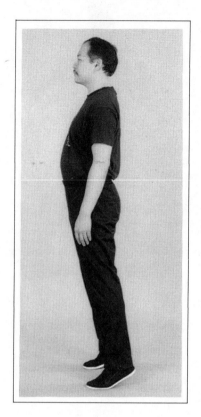

Beginning with your feet close together and arms relaxed at your sides, straighten your legs and slowly lift your heels high off the ground and hold for three seconds. Slowly lower yourself back to starting position. Repeat eight times.

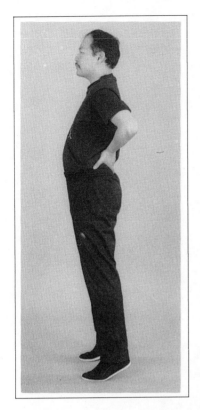

Place your hands on your back as shown and repeat raising and lowering your heels eight times.

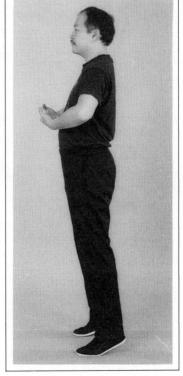

With your fingers pointing inward and palms facing upward, again repeat raising and lowering heels, eight times.

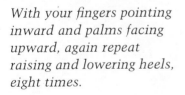

3. Balances heart channel

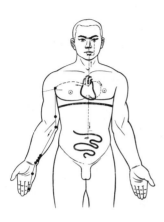

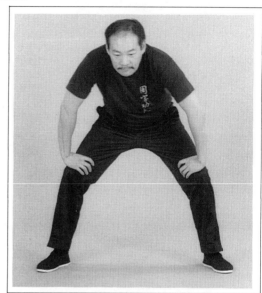

*With your legs
wider than
shoulder-width
apart, place your
palms on your
thighs with
thumbs on the
inside of each leg.*

*Turn and slowly
bend as far to the
right as possible
without raising your
feet off the ground.
Hold for three
seconds.*

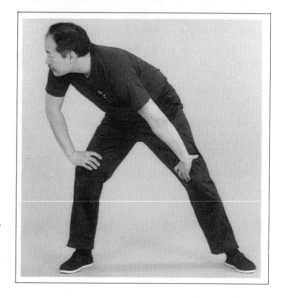

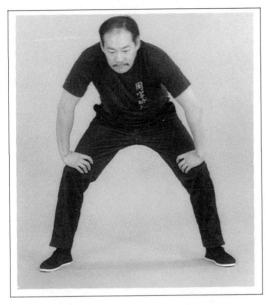

Return to the starting position and repeat to the left. Repeat the exercise twelve times on each side.

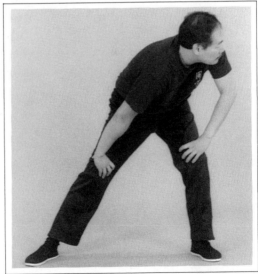

4. Balances kidney channel

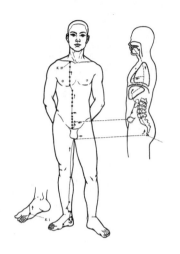

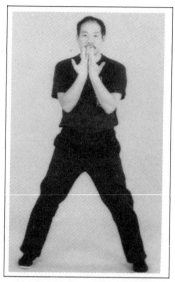

Start with your legs wider than shoulder-width apart and slightly bent. With the backs of your hands pressed together, raise your arms up to chest level.

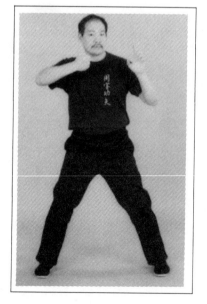

As you turn to the left, extend your left arm as shown and draw back your right fist . . .

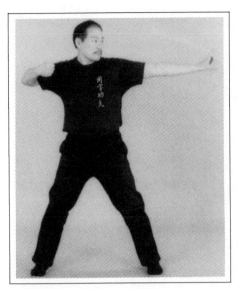

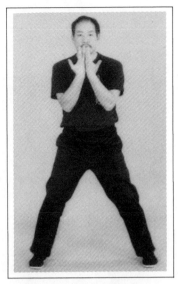

. . . as if drawing an arrow in a bow. Hold for three seconds.

Slowly return to the starting position.

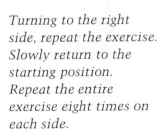

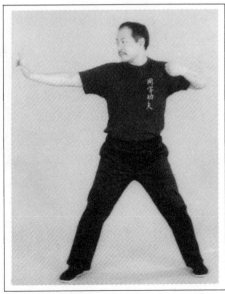

Turning to the right side, repeat the exercise. Slowly return to the starting position. Repeat the entire exercise eight times on each side.

5. Balances all channels

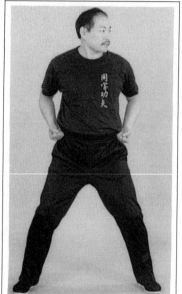

Starting with your legs bent and wider than shoulder-width apart, hold both fists at your sides as shown.

While turning to face left, extend your left arm to the side with your palm open. Hold for three seconds.

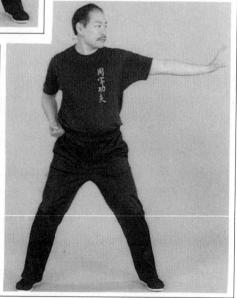

*Repeat to the right and
return to the starting
position. Repeat exercise
twelve times on each side.*

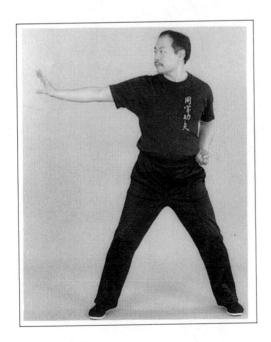

6. *Balances stomach, spleen, and liver channels*

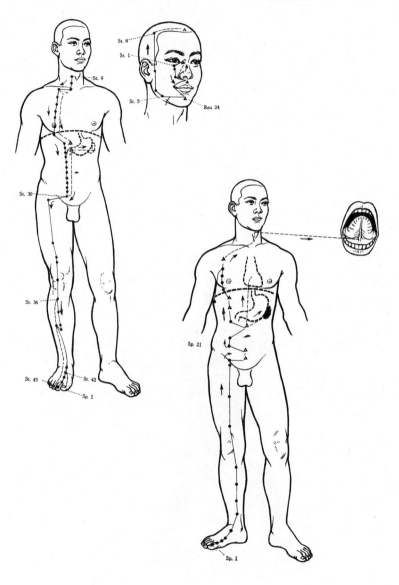

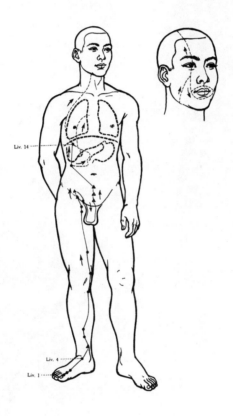

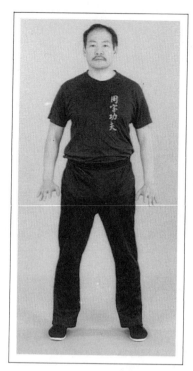

Begin with your body in a natural stance, palms facing downward, fingers pointing forward.

Cross your arms with the right arm on the outside and raise to stomach level.

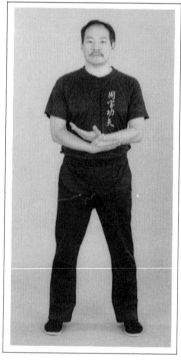

As your right arm continues upward with the palm facing up, extend your left arm downward with the palm parallel to the floor.

Extend your arms until the right arm is directly overhead, palm up and pointed inward, and the left arm is at your side, fingers pointing forward, palm facing down. Hold for three seconds.

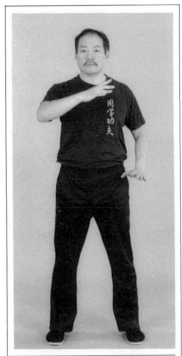

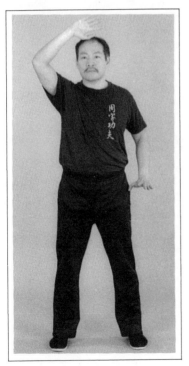

Slowly reverse the movement to change arms, with your left arm crossing on the outside. Repeat the extension on the opposite side and hold for three seconds. Repeat the exercise a total of twelve times on each side.

7. Balances triple channel

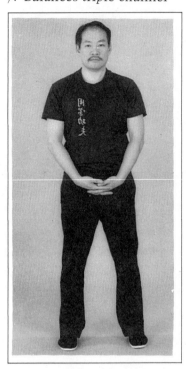

Slowly raise your arms overhead with palms facing toward your chest on the way up, and upward when hands are over your head.

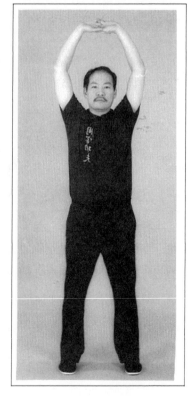

Intertwine your fingers with your palms facing upward.

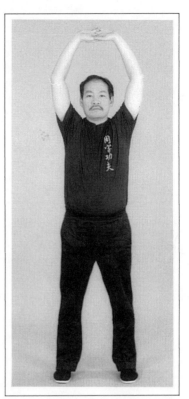

While holding your arms overhead, slowly lean as far to the right as possible.

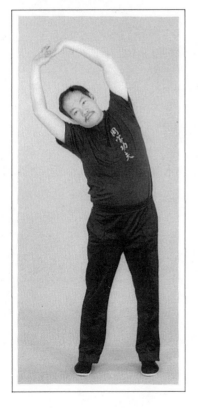

Return to the center. Now lean to the left as far as possible and return to the center. Repeat exercise a total of twelve times on each side.

8. Balances kidney channel

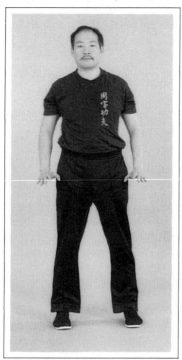

Begin with your arms at your sides, palms facing downward, fingers forward.

Raise your arms so that your fingers point inward and your palms face inward.

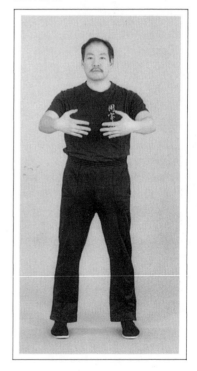

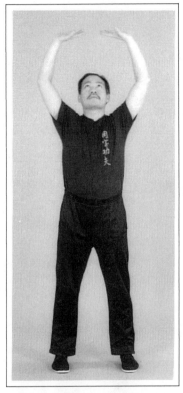

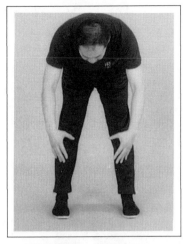

Still holding your arms overhead, slowly bend forward at the waist.

Continue moving downward until you reach the floor. Hold your toes or ankles for three seconds.

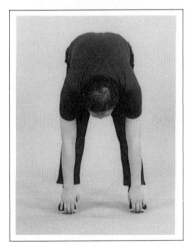

Looking upward, raise your arms overhead, palms facing upward, and hold for three seconds.

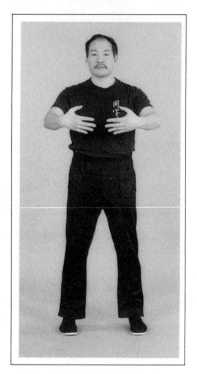

Slowly return to a standing position with your palms facing inward.

Return to the starting position with your palms facing downward at your sides. Repeat the entire series of movements twelve times.

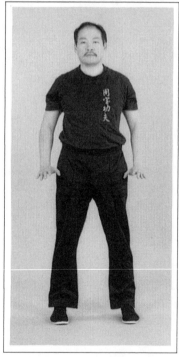

Now that you are familiar with each part of the thirty-day energetic workout, you are ready to begin. First study the worksheet on page 196. Do *only* the exercises listed for each day of the program. Even if you are flexible and in good overall physical condition, the level of mental concentration that must accompany each exercise must be raised slowly in order to be effective. You must give yourself time to commit each one to memory. Some of you may find it helpful to create your own audiotape of these exercises by slowly reading the exercise instructions into a tape recorder (be sure to leave yourself enough time to perform the movements by pausing between instructions). Once you have familiarized yourself with the correct position from these photos, you can run through each exercise using your tape to guide you, and in this way avoid interrupting your routine to consult the book.

Before you begin:

- Follow each direction carefully.
- Begin each exercise with a calm mind and proper posture.
- Make sure you are breathing correctly and consistently throughout each exercise.
- Concentrate on feeling your energy. Move slowly. Your physical movements will slow down naturally when you increase your mental concentration, but until then, you must make sure each exercise is performed with strong mental focus.
- Commit yourself to increasing your energy. Once you decide to begin the thirty-day energetic work-

out, don't stop until you have completed the program. Develop the patience you need to maximize your energy.

You should start realizing results within a few days. After thirty days of following this program, along with the other guidelines contained in this book, you should look better, feel better, and have a lot more energy to bring to every part of your life.

THIRTY-DAY ENERGETIC WORKOUT

	Exercise	Approx. Workout Running Time	Check When Done
Day 1	Stretching only	5 minutes	_____
Day 2	Stretching only	5 minutes	_____
Day 3	Stretching only	5 minutes	_____
Day 4	Stretching, exercise 1	8 minutes	_____
Day 5	Stretching, exercise 1	8 minutes	_____
Day 6	Stretching, exercise 1	8 minutes	_____
Day 7	Stretching, exercises 1 and 2	11 minutes	_____
Day 8	Stretching, exercises 1 and 2	11 minutes	_____
Day 9	Stretching, exercises 1 and 2	11 minutes	_____
Day 10	Stretching, exercises 1–3	14 minutes	_____
Day 11	Stretching, exercises 1–3	14 minutes	_____
Day 12	Stretching, exercises 1–3	14 minutes	_____
Day 13	Stretching, exercises 1–4	17 minutes	_____
Day 14	Stretching, exercises 1–4	17 minutes	_____
Day 15	Stretching, exercises 1–4	17 minutes	_____
Day 16	Advanced stretching, exercises 1–4	18 minutes	_____

THIRTY-DAY ENERGETIC WORKOUT (*Continued*)

	Exercise	Approx. Workout Running Time	Check When Done
Day 17	Advanced stretching, exercises 1–4	18 minutes	_____
Day 18	Advanced stretching, exercises 1–4	18 minutes	_____
Day 19	Advanced stretching, exercises 1–5	21 minutes	_____
Day 20	Advanced stretching, exercises 1–5	21 minutes	_____
Day 21	Advanced stretching, exercises 1–5	21 minutes	_____
Day 22	Advanced stretching, exercises 1–6	24 minutes	_____
Day 23	Advanced stretching, exercises 1–6	24 minutes	_____
Day 24	Advanced stretching, exercises 1–6	24 minutes	_____
Day 25	Advanced stretching, exercises 1–7	27 minutes	_____
Day 26	Advanced stretching, exercises 1–7	27 minutes	_____
Day 27	Advanced stretching, exercises 1–7	27 minutes	_____
Day 28	Advanced stretching, exercises 1–8	30 minutes	_____
Day 29	Advanced stretching, exercises 1–8	30 minutes	_____
Day 30	Advanced stretching, exercises 1–8	30 minutes	_____

* On Day 16, add the two advanced stretches illustrated in figures 26, 28, and 29.

AFTERWORD

CONGRATULATIONS ON completing the thirty-day energetic workout. Now that you have made a commitment to developing your own inner energy, you have changed your life forever. If you have not been able to memorize the entire program, continue working to do so. This way you will have a powerful energy-building and balancing tool to carry with you wherever you go.

You should already look and feel better. But this is only the beginning. Continue to perform the workout as often as possible. If you simply want to maintain the new level of energy in your life, do the workout three times per week. But if you want to keep increasing your energy, continue to practice it daily. Within six months of continued practice you should feel a dramatic increase in your energy level. And you can further increase your energy by doing each exercise longer. You can also further develop your energetic power by studying tai chi, yoga, or a martial art. At the very least, whenever you need a quick, five-minute "energy pickup," just do each of the eight exercises for less than a minute—instead of reaching for a cup of coffee. You'll be amazed by how just a little effort yields immediate results once you are in touch with your own energy.

I hope this book has helped you "realize" your own energy. The time you invest in developing your inner energy will provide you with many benefits throughout your life. Energetic masters who routinely perform "miracles," whether healing others or themselves, generally exercise daily for up to three hours. Just like them, your energy potential is only limited by the amount of hard work and determination you put into it. You alone control your inner energy—and your inner energy is the underlying essence of your life. Use it to unlock your life's full potential.

APPENDIX

The American Association of Acupuncture
and Oriental Medicine
1424 16th Street, NW, Suite 501
Washington, D.C. 20036
(202) 265-2287

The Q.M. Institute—Headquarters
121 East 37th Street, Suite 4B
New York, New York 10016
(212) 765-6729

Osaka Center for Oriental Therapy
50 West 56th Street
New York, New York 10019
(212) 682-1779

Q.M. Institute branch offices are located at:

300 West 55th Street, Suite 7D
New York, New York 10019

5 Richards Avenue
Dover, New Jersey 07801

ABOUT THE AUTHOR

AN ACUPUNCTURE physician trained in both Western and Eastern medicine, martial arts world champion, and author, Dr. Richard M. Chin has dedicated much of the past twenty-five years to introducing acupuncture, martial arts, and other aspects of Eastern culture to the Western world. His efforts have been featured in magazines including *Town & Country*, *The New Yorker*, *Lear's*, and *Self*, as well as on the Fox Television program *A Current Affair* and ABC's *A.M. New York*.

A master of the martial arts jow ga kung fu, bok mei, and tai chi chuan, Dr. Chin also holds an eighth degree black belt in shai jow kung fu. He is the founder and president of the Asian Martial Arts Association and coauthor, with Susan Ribner, of the classic text *The Martial Arts*.

Dr. Chin holds O.M.D. degrees from both the California Acupuncture College in Los Angeles and the Chinese Research Center in Hong Kong. He also holds an M.D. degree from Far Eastern University in the Philippines. Dr. Chin is a former member of the board of directors of the American Association of Acupuncture and Oriental Medicine (AAAOM), and was formerly the International Representative of the National Commission for Certification of Acupuncturists (NCCA). He is the founder and director of the Q.M. Institute in Manhattan, one of the first clinics in New York to combine Eastern and Western medical practices.